Electrical Impedance Tomography

The Adam Hilger Series on Biomedical Engineering

Series Editor: **J G Webster**

The Adam Hilger Series on Biomedical Engineering

Electrical Impedance Tomography

Edited by

J G Webster

Department of Electrical and Computer Engineering, University of Wisconsin–Madison

Adam Hilger, Bristol and New York

British Library Cataloguing in Publication Data

Electrical impedance tomography.
1. an. Diagnosis. Tomography
I. Webster, J. G.
616.0757

ISBN 0-85274-304-1

Library of Congress Cataloging-in-Publication Data are available

The author has attempted to trace the copyright holder of all the figures reproduced in this publication and apologizes to copyright holders if permission to publish in this form has not been obtained.

Published under the Adam Hilger imprint by IOP Publishing Ltd
Techno House, Redcliffe Way, Bristol BS1 6NX, England
335 East 45th Street, New York, NY 10017-3483, USA

Printed in Great Britain by Galliard (Printers) Ltd, Great Yarmouth, Norfolk

Contents

Preface

Electrical impedance measurements contribute to medical care. Two-electrode infant apnea monitors yield a measure of the depth of ventilation. Four-electrode impedance cardiographs yield a measure of cardiac output. Other electrical impedance measurements have been demonstrated in research laboratories, but few have proven useful in clinical practice.

Will electrical impedance tomography be useful in clinical practice? To answer this question, we must construct complex instruments, practical electrode arrays and sophisticated reconstruction algorithms. We must prove they yield reasonable images on saline-filled physical phantoms. Then we must obtain useful results from tests on animals and humans. Finally physicians must tell us, 'Yes, this method provides me information on my patients better than the method I am using now' Until all of these tasks have been accomplished, our task is not done. We must peform much research before we can answer the question.

This book includes information to begin the research. Chapter 1 reviews the present competing imaging methods, presents a short history of electrical impedance imaging, and touches on some of the major problems. Chapter 2 describes tissue resistivity—the very thing we are trying to distinguish—and shows that we cannot ignore the skin impedance in our computer models.

I believe electrodes will be one of our major problems. Chapter 3 describes the variety of electrodes available. But the biggest problem is that we cannot locate them precisely on our irregularly shaped body. And if the computer does not know precisely where the electrodes are, it has difficulty reconstructing static images.

Chapters 4 and 5 cover instrument design. Current generators require driven shields to maintain high output impedance and high amplitude stability. We must design switching matrices and voltage amplifiers to prevent errors due to attenuation and phase shift. Demodulators and filters must keep the ripple low, yet respond quickly to switching transients. Chapter 6 describes electrical safety and the barriers that must exist within the circuits to prevent excessive current from harming the patient.

Chapter 7 describes the required computer size. To achieve adequate spatial resolution, we require many pixels (picture elements). But to invert the resulting matrices requires days or weeks on a small computer. The use of a supercomputer is an expensive solution now.

Early workers injected current through all possible electrodes. Chapter 8 describes the simplifying trend to injecting current through only two electrodes. Now the most promising data collection method is the adaptive method, which injects currents through all electrodes in a way that optimizes the ability to distinguish resistivity differences. Chapter 9 describes errors caused by electrode location, stray capacitance, quantization and contact impedance.

Chapter 10 demonstrates that there are many possible reconstruction algorithms. Some are simple, fast, but inaccurate. Others are more accurate, but take a long time, or require perfect data. Those who can demonstrate impressive images from computer models should realize that the goal of demonstrating static images from humans will require algorithms that can tolerate considerable error in the collected data. Chapter 11 describes the computational complexity of these algorithms, with emphasis on finite element methods and simplification of sparse matrices. Chapter 12 discusses several measures of performance, including spatial resolution, conductivity contrast, conductivity resolution, distinguishability, and temporal resolution.

If we cannot find an application for electrical impedance imaging, then the work is not practical. Chapter 13 lists the many applications that have been proposed. For each it mentions the way measurements are made now, and how it might be possible to use electrical impedance tomography. All of these are possibilities, but none of them shows any clear advantage now. Yet I have the intuitive feeling that the advantage may be there, if not for obtaining an image, then at least for obtaining one-dimensional measurements. For example, infant apnea monitors presently use two electrodes, but have major problems with motion artifacts. I believe 4 to 16 electrodes arranged in a polka-dot pattern around the chest could measure ventilation with a better signal-to-artifact ratio.

Chapter 14 covers geophysical prospecting, where the four-electrode method is most common. The additional number of electrodes used by electrical impedance tomography might improve the ability to locate subterranean ore bodies. Chapter 15 lists active groups and companies and should assist in communicating with each other. All the references are collected alphabetically in Chapter 16.

Someday a useful result may come from the research described here. I hope that this book will play a part in suggesting the hardware and software development to achieve the goal of a practical clinical instrument. I would welcome your suggestions for improvement of future editions.

John G Webster
Madison, Wisconsin
December 1989

1

Electrical Impedance Imaging

John G Webster

This chapter describes instruments that form images of electric resistivity or conductivity within the body. It begins with a technique that yields a frontal plane image by applying a checkerboard array of electrodes on the back. It presents the development of instruments that yield a cross-sectional image in the manner of computed tomography. It also presents the few efforts to present a three-dimensional distribution of resistivity in the body and describes the difference between static and dynamic imaging. A brief description of the hardware surveys the current injecting and voltage measuring systems.

1.1 IMAGING METHODS

1.1.1 X-ray imaging

The most common medical imaging technique uses X rays. X rays travel in straight lines through the body and cause darkening of photographic film behind the body. X rays traveling though bone are attenuated and yield less film darkening. X-ray films have excellent spatial resolution. However, X rays are damaging to tissue and can cause cancer.

1.1.2 Computerized tomography (CT)

In computerized tomography, a pencil-like beam of X rays passes through the body to detectors from all angles in a plane. A computer uses the resulting attenuation data to calculate the two-dimensional image in the plane. The instrument has excellent spatial resolution, but is large and expensive.

1.1.3 Gamma camera

Gamma cameras provide an image of organ function. Radiopharmaceuticals are introduced into the body and concentrate in target organs. As they undergo radioactive decay, they emit gamma rays, which cause light flashes in a nearby scintillation crystal. Photodetectors yield a fuzzy image of the concentration of the radiopharmaceutical. The dose is kept small to avoid damage from the radiation.

1.1.4 Magnetic resonance imaging (MRI)

Magnetic resonance imaging images the distribution of certain chemicals, such as the hydrogen in water. The patient is placed in a strong magnetic field. The precessing of the hydrogen atoms is scanned with an oscillating electric field to yield the distribution with excellent spatial resolution. The instrument is very large and expensive, but there is no damage to the patient.

1.1.5 Ultrasonic imaging

In ultrasonic imaging, a beam of ultrasound passes from a transducer into the body, and is reflected from internal organs. The amplitude, distance, and angle of reflected ultrasound are collected by the transducer and processed to yield the image. The instrument is reasonable in cost and is nondamaging to tissue.

1.2 FRONTAL PLANE IMPEDANCE IMAGING

1.2.1 Instrument design

Even as X rays travel from the front to the back of the chest, electric currents can travel from the front to the back of the chest. Swanson (1976) proposed the first frontal plane impedance imaging technique. Henderson *et al* (1976) and Henderson and Webster (1978) designed the impedance camera shown in figure 1.1. They applied a constant 100 kHz voltage to a large electrode on the chest, which resulted in varying currents collected through a 100-electrode array on the back. All electrodes except for the measuring electrode were maintained at 0 V, which resulted in a large guard electrode around the measuring electrode.

1.2.2 Frontal plane images

Figure 1.2 shows the resulting image, which shows variations in admittance of each electrode from 250 to 650 μS. The low admittances occurred over each lung because the lung tissue has low conductivity. However, the image is certainly crude and distorted because, unlike X rays, electric currents do not travel in straight lines. Thus they suggested the use of computerized tomography reconstruction techniques.

1.3 TRANSVERSE PLANE IMPEDANCE IMAGING

1.3.1 Parallel current lines

Lytle and Dines (1978) simulated a square computer model of a two-dimensional transverse plane. For each angle, they varied the voltage on all electrodes to achieve parallel current lines in a homogeneous medium. Then they used these voltage distributions when simulated objects were inside and calculated the resulting currents. From this data set, they reconstructed the image by solving Laplace's equation and computed the resistivity profile by back projection in about 10 iterations.

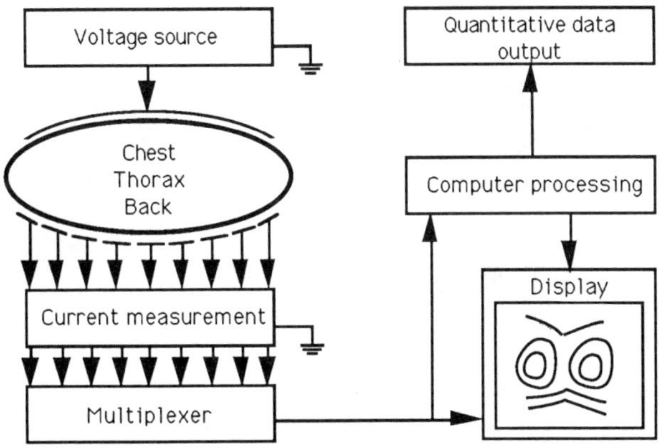

Figure 1.1 The frontal plane impedance camera applied voltage to one large electrode on the chest and measured current from each of 100 electrodes on the back (Henderson and Webster 1978).

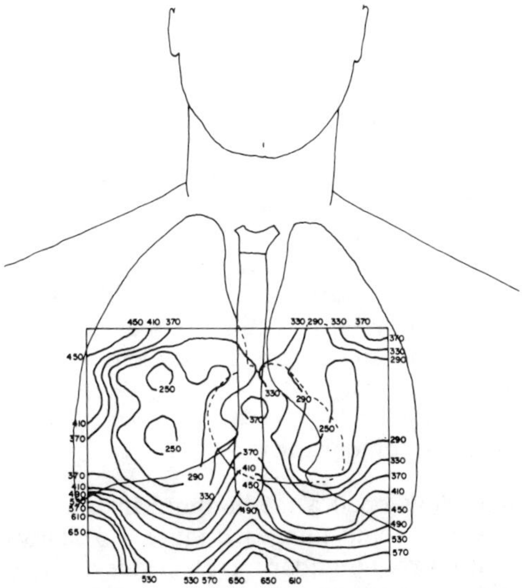

Figure 1.2 Isoadmittance contour map of human thorax. Admittance values are in microsiemens per electrode (Henderson and Webster 1978).

1.3.2 Finite difference method

Tasto and Schomberg (1978) simulated a square computer model of a two-dimensional transverse plane. For from 1 to 432 projection angles, they determined the voltage distribution for each projection angle using the two-dimensional finite difference method and the overrelaxation technique. Figure 1.3 shows their success in reconstructing a difficult object.

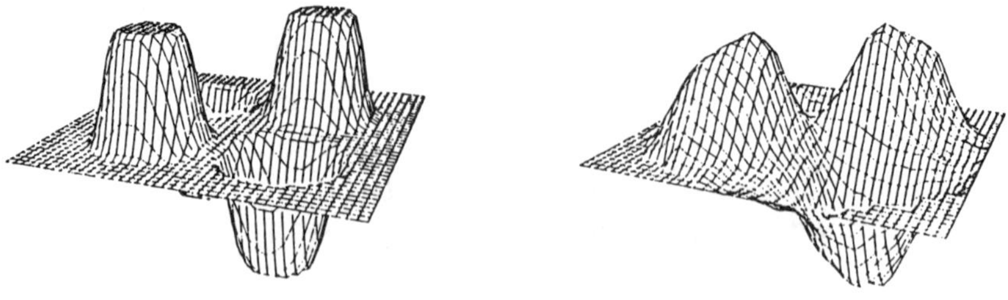

Original object   Reconstructed object

Figure 1.3 Original and reconstructed object with no rotational symmetry (Tasto and Schomberg 1978).

1.3.3 Perturbation method

Kim *et al* (1983) simulated a circular computer model of a two-dimensional transverse plane. For a constant voltage input, they changed the resistivity of each picture element (pixel) and measured the resulting current changes in all electrodes. They used the resulting perturbation matrix and Laplace's equation to backproject differences between true and computed current densities according to each element's sensitivity to each electrode. The model used 332 elements, four projection angles, the finite element method, and about 200 iterations to reconstruct an image.

1.3.4 Applied potential tomography

Barber *et al* (1983) developed a method and instrument for obtaining two-dimensional transverse plane images. Figure 1.4 shows that they injected 50 kHz current into two neighboring electrodes. They assumed that the resistivity was uniform and calculated the expected voltages between all other pairs of electrodes. If the measured voltage on a real object was high by some factor, they multiplied the model resistivity by that factor everywhere in the shaded region. They repeated for all possible voltage measurements for all possible current injections and averaged all the results. While the spatial resolution is poorer than other methods, the method is so fast that they can take 20 samples/s and image changes during a cardiac cycle.

1.3.5 Adaptive currents

Gisser *et al* (1987) simulated a circular model of a two-dimensional transverse plane. Instead of constraining the current to only two or a limited number of

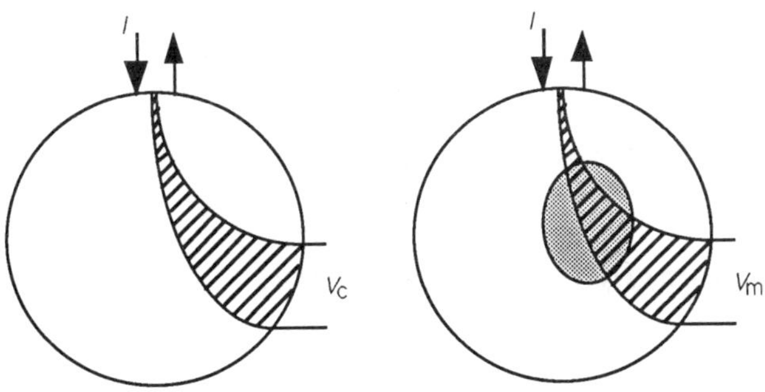

Figure 1.4 If the measured voltage is higher than the calculated voltage, multiply the resistivity in the shaded area by that factor (Barber *et al* 1983).

electrodes, they placed current on all electrodes. They developed a method for automatically adapting the current distribution to optimize distinguishability of internal objects. For example, for a central object, the optimal current distribution is $\cos n\theta$, where θ is the angle around the circular model. The higher current density obtained through the object increases its distinguishability.

1.4 THREE-DIMENSIONAL IMPEDANCE IMAGING

1.4.1 Measurements from the surface

Wexler *et al* (1985) simulated a cubic model of a three-dimensional solid. The model contains four layers of 7×7 volume elements (voxels). Because they were interested in geophysical prospecting, they permitted measurements at the top surface only. They demonstrated fair reconstruction of an object in layers 2 and 3 whose conductivity was five times that of the host medium in 1700 iterations.

1.4.2 Measurements from the sides

Liu *et al* (1988) simulated a cubic model of a three-dimensional solid. The model contained three layers of 4×4 voxels. Because they were interested in imaging the thorax, they permitted measurements at the sides only. They obtained superior results when electrodes were placed in a diagonal between two planes than when they were in only one plane. They were able to successfully image up to 18 objects at random locations in three iterations.

1.4.3 Recent three-dimensional work

Goble and Isaacson (1989) constructed a three-dimensional saline tank phantom with 64 electrodes. The phantom had four layers of electrodes and each layer had 16 equidistantly placed stainless steel electrodes. They used an algorithm which computed optimal patterns of injection current in three dimensions and studied the effects of electrode geometry, target volume and target height on distinguishability. They reported that the stacked cosine patterns of injection current maximize distinguishability for cylindrical targets centered in the phantom. Ider *et al* (1989) developed an algorithm for compensating three-dimensional effects in EIT based on the assumption that the objects are finite cylindrical structures with a translationally uniform impedance distribution. They argued that the compensation algorithm could be applied to impedance imaging of limbs and to a lesser extent the thorax.

1.5 STATIC VERSUS DYNAMIC IMAGING

1.5.1 Static imaging

We desire to obtain static images of resistivity distribution. All computer simulations perform static images easily because they use perfect data obtained from perfect coordinate systems. Thus any results obtained from computer simulations are deceiving. When data are obtained from real electrodes on real bodies, the measured data have location errors that prevent reconstruction of images. Barber *et al* (1983) found that they could not locate electrodes accurately enough, even when placed in a rigid ring. Also, placing electrodes on the noncircular thorax added additional location errors. It is possible that the lower spatial frequencies used by Gisser *et al* (1987) may ease the problem somewhat, but that remains to be demonstrated.

1.5.2 Dynamic imaging

Dynamic imaging means taking reference data at time 1, then modified data at time 2, then processing these data to obtain a difference image. Thus Barber *et al* (1983) used electrodes in a rigid ring to obtain data 1 from an isotropic bath of saline. Then they put the ring around the forearm and took data 2. By subtracting these they obtained a difference image that looks like a static image—but it is not. They found it not possible to apply electrodes to a body and obtain a static image.

Dynamic images can be useful. Barber *et al* (1983) take a rubber band marked at 16 evenly spaced intervals and stretch it around the chest. They place a disposable ECG electrode at each location. They take difference images at different times in the breathing or cardiac cycles and display their effects. They can drink water and obtain images of stomach emptying. They can monitor temperature rise during hyperthermia treatment for cancer.

Griffiths and Ahmed (1987a) suggest one possible way to obtain a static image. They obtain images using data at two different frequencies of 100 kHz and 150 kHz in a computer simulation. However, the difference image was very different from a static image.

1.6 ELECTRICAL IMPEDANCE TOMOGRAPHY HARDWARE

An electrical impedance tomography instrument has one or more current sources that inject AC current into an object—such as the body. Figure 1.5

shows that the current sources require a control circuit. A single current source requires switches that direct it into many different electrode combinations. Multiple current sources require a control circuit that adjusts the magnitude of each current source to achieve desired patterns of current density.

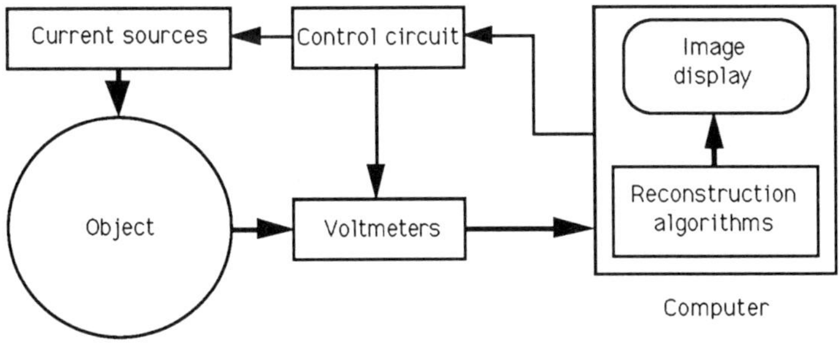

Figure 1.5 An electrical impedance tomography system injects currents into an object and measures voltages from it.

A single voltmeter consists of a differential amplifier, a phase-sensitive demodulator, a low-pass filter, and switches that measure from many different electrode combinations. Multiple voltmeters can operate in parallel to speed data acquisition time. After the data are in the computer, reconstruction algorithms process them to display the image of the resistivity distribution in the object.

1.7 STUDY QUESTIONS

1.1 For frontal plane imaging, show the circuit design for a current-to-voltage converter.
1.2 For frontal plane imaging, show the switching required so every unused electrode is held at ground potential.
1.3 Describe the electrode voltage distribution used by Lytle and Dynes.
1.4 Explain how dynamic imaging differs from static imaging and why Barber *et al* could not obtain static images.
1.5 Describe the electrode voltage distribution used by Wexler *et al* and the number of voxels in their computer model.
1.6 Describe the electrode voltage distribution used by Liu *et al* and the number of voxels in their computer model.
1.7 Describe the electrode current distribution used by Gisser *et al* and list the differences between it and that used by others.

2

Tissue Resistivity

Ammar Rabbat

In this chapter we present the equivalent electric circuit models of tissues. We explain the dependence of tissue impedance on electric parameters, such as the resistivity and permittivity. We describe the different factors that influence the impedance of tissues. These factors are: frequency, time, temperature, and directional placement. Finally, we collect data on impedances of mammalian organ impedances.

2.1 TISSUE CHARACTERISTICS

Figure 2.1 shows the basic structure of tissue, which consists of an aggregate of cells surrounded by fluids. Each cell is surrounded by a membrane that envelops intracellular fluids. At low frequencies, the cellular membrane has a high resistance and, therefore, the current travels through the extracellular fluids around the cells (bold lines). At high frequencies, the capacitance of the cellular membrane short circuits the resistance of the membrane. Then the current lines pass uniformly through the tissue structure (fine lines). Figure 2.2 shows that the impedance of tissue decreases with frequency because of this short circuiting of the cellular membrane resistance.

2.2 ELECTRIC CIRCUIT MODELS OF IMPEDANCE

2.2.1 Electric circuit models

Tissues consist of cells and fluids. Figure 2.3 shows that each cell is surrounded by a membrane that envelops the intracellular fluids. A membrane is an ultrathin (6 nm) highly resistive layer that can be electrically modeled as a capacitance (C_m) in parallel with a resistance (R_m). The intracellular fluids can be modeled as a resistance (R_i). The extracellular fluids can also be modeled as a resistance (R_e). This model can be simplified to the four-element model (figure 2.4(*a*)) and further simplified to the three-element model (figure 2.4(*b*)).

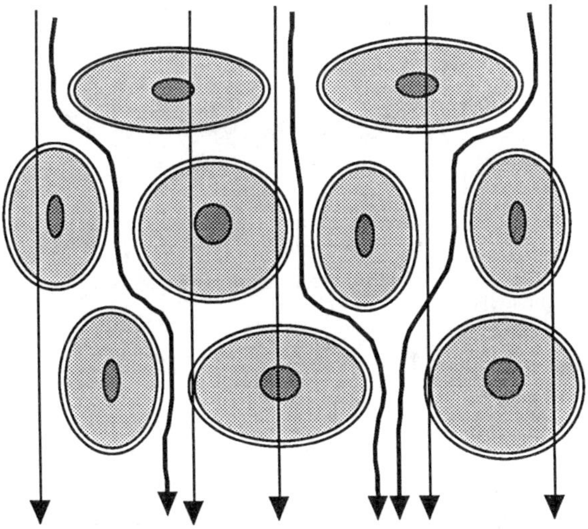

Figure 2.1 At high frequencies, the cell membrane is short circuited and the current travels in straight (thin) lines. At low frequencies, the current travels longer paths through only the extracellular fluid (bold lines).

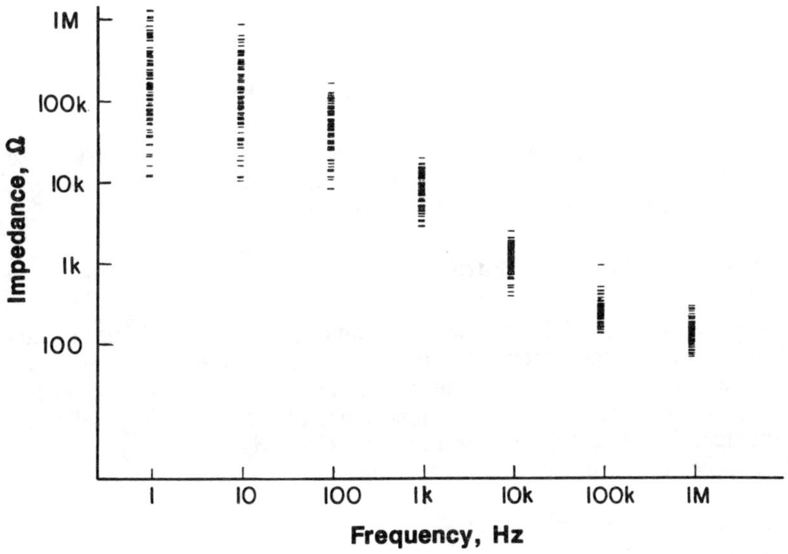

Figure 2.2 The impedance of 1 cm^2 of unabraded skin decreases with frequency (Rosell *et al* 1988a).

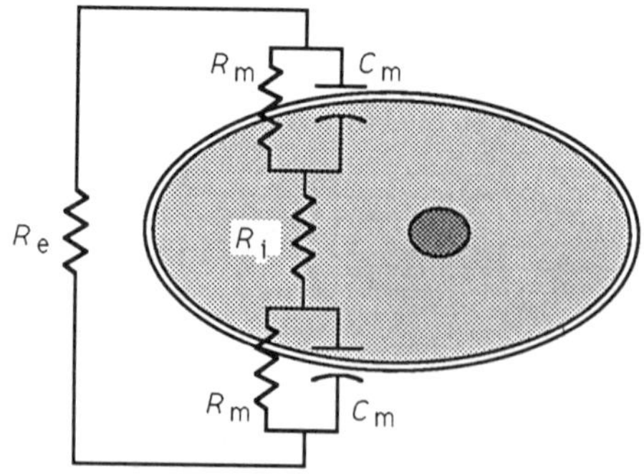

Figure 2.3 Current can travel through the cell membrane and also through the extracellular resistance between the cells.

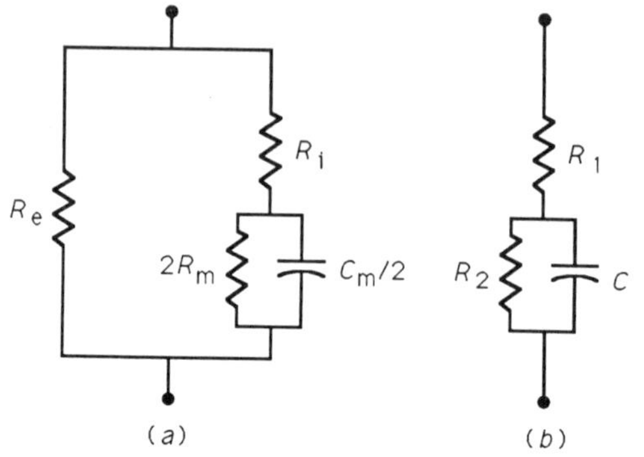

Figure 2.4 The (*a*) four- and (*b*) three-element models of tissue.

We can also model tissues with a distributed circuit which consists of series *R–C* elements with many parallel branches. Kanai *et al* (1987) described and derived equations for a distributed model for tissues.

2.2.2 Conductivity and permittivity

The electric circuit models (figures 2.4(*a*) and (*b*)) show that tissue impedance is complex. For the measurement of this impedance, one of two representations is used: a complex series impedance (resistance in series with a reactance, figure 2.5(*a*)) or a complex parallel admittance (conductance in parallel with a capacitance, figure 2.5(*b*)). We will use the following terminology to describe the two impedance representations (Schwan 1957).

The complex series impedance:
R is the resistance (Ω)
X is the reactance (Ω)
$Z = R + jX$ is the impedance (Ω)

The complex parallel admittance:

G is the conductance (S)
C is the capacitance (F)
$Y = G + j\omega C$ is the admittance (S)

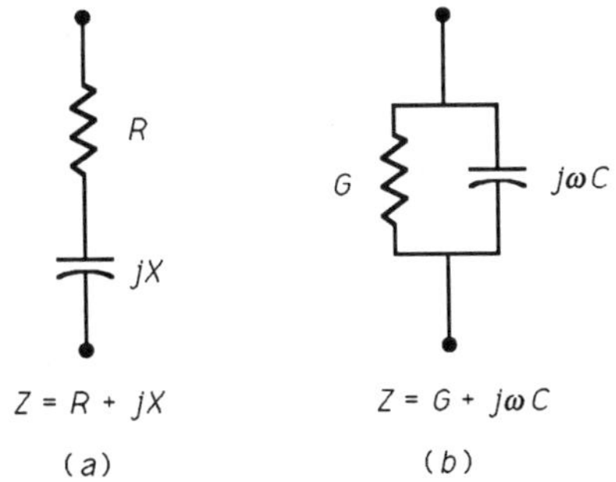

Figure 2.5 The (*a*) series and (*b*) parallel representations of complex impedance.

We can use the following equation to convert the admittance to the impedance:

$$Z = \frac{1}{Y} \tag{2.1}$$

$$R + jX = \frac{1}{G + j\omega C} \tag{2.2}$$

$$R = \frac{G}{G^2 + \omega^2 C^2} \tag{2.3}$$

$$X = \frac{-\omega C}{G^2 + \omega^2 C^2}. \tag{2.4}$$

Many scientists have measured the tissue impedance in terms of the conductivity and permittivity. Equations (2.5) to (2.8) show the relation between the complex impedance and the conductivity σ and permittivity ε,

$$C = \frac{\varepsilon\varepsilon_0 A}{d} \text{ (F)} \tag{2.5}$$

$$G = \frac{\sigma A}{d} \text{ (S)} \tag{2.6}$$

$$Y = G + j\omega C = \frac{(\sigma + j\omega\varepsilon\varepsilon_0)A}{d} \tag{2.7}$$

$$Z = 1/Y = \frac{d}{(\sigma + j\omega\varepsilon\varepsilon_0)A} \tag{2.8}$$

where A is the area of the specimen (m^2), d is the depth of the specimen (m), σ is the conductivity (S/m), ε is the relative permittivity (dielectric constant), ε_0 is the permittivity of vacuum (8.85×10^{-12} (F/m)), and $\omega = 2\pi f$.

Note that the permittivity of tissue is a representation of the dielectric properties of the complete tissue structure and is not a representation of a specific physical substance. This is because the tissue relative permittivity can be as high as 3×10^6 (figure 2.6) where the relative permittivity of physical substances range from a value close to 1 for gases to a maximum of 300 for solids.

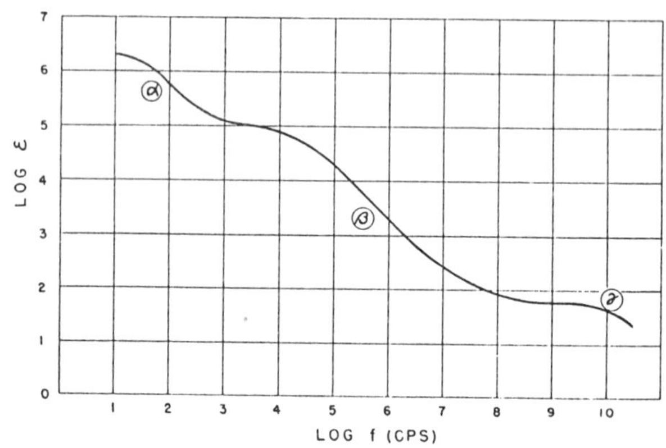

Figure 2.6 The dielectric constant for muscular tissue decreases with frequency (Schwan 1957).

2.2.3 Cole–Cole plot

The complex series impedance ($R + jX$) can be represented by a plot of the real component R versus the imaginary component X for the impedance at different frequencies. This plot is commonly called a Cole–Cole plot (Cole and Cole 1941). Figure 2.7 shows the Cole–Cole plot of an impedance with a single time constant which is given by the following equation:

$$Z = R_\infty + \frac{R_0 - R_\infty}{1 + j\omega\tau} \tag{2.9}$$

where R_0 is the resistance at $f = 0$, R_∞ is the resistance at $f = \infty$, and τ is the time constant.

The plot is a semicircle of a radius equal to $(R_0 - R_\infty)/2$ and intercepts the real axis at R_0 and R_∞. The total impedance (Z_t) of the three-element circuit presented in figure 2.4(b) is an example of an impedance with a single time constant where: $R_0 = R_1 + R_2$, $R_\infty = R_1$, and $\tau = R_2 C$.

The complex series impedance of tissues is commonly represented by a Cole–Cole plot. However, in practice, data measured on most tissues fit a semicircle with a center that is depressed below the real axis (figure 2.8). Cole and Cole (1941) noted that the depressed semicircular locus is a representation of an impedance of the form given in equation (2.9) and the depression angle ϕ is equal to $(1 - \alpha)\pi/2$,

$$Z = R_\infty + \frac{R_0 - R_\infty}{1 + (j\omega\tau)^{(1-\alpha)}}. \tag{2.10}$$

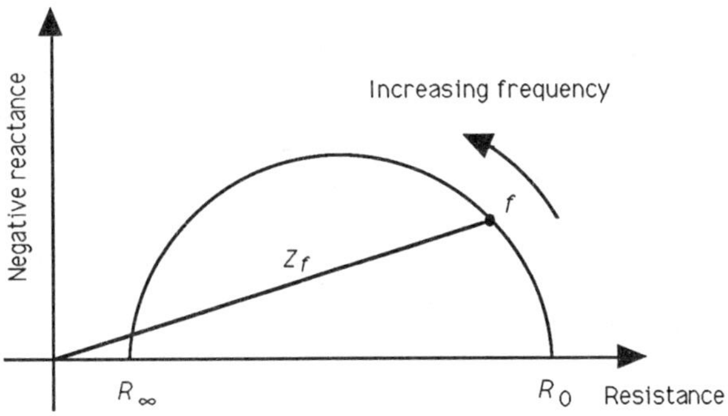

Figure 2.7 The Cole–Cole plot for impedance with a single time constant.

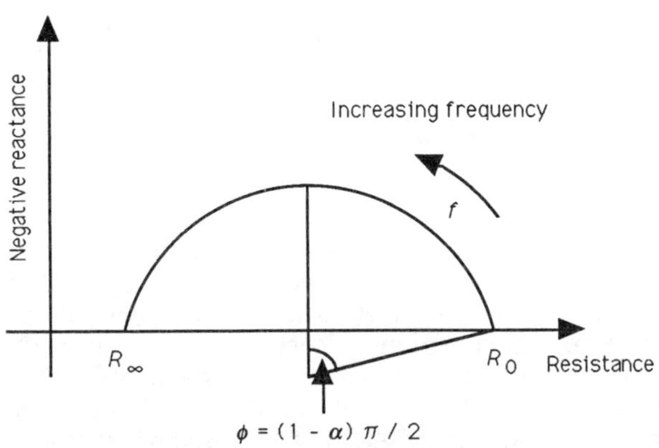

Figure 2.8 The depressed Cole–Cole plot.

2.3 CELLULAR ELECTRICAL PROPERTIES

The cell is the basic building component of tissues. It consists of a membrane surrounding the intracellular fluid, the cytoplasm. Membranes are ultrathin layers with a thickness of the order of 6 nm and are composed mainly of lipids and proteins and smaller amounts of other substances such as water and sugar (Pethig 1979). The functioning of the membrane depends on the relative amounts of the lipid and protein components. Pethig (1979) showed that proteins make up 51% of the membrane and lipids make up 47%. The membrane is highly resistive and has the electrical characteristics of a capacitance in parallel with a resistance (C_m and R_m in figure 2.3). Pethig (1984) reported values for the membrane capacitance from 0.5 to 1.3 μF/cm^2 with a typical value of 1 μF/cm^2 (this can be multiplied by area to obtain membrane capacitance). He also reported values for the membrane resistance that range from 100 Ω cm^2 to 100 kΩ cm^2 (this can be divided by area to obtain tissue resistance). The resistivity of the intracellular fluids is 60 Ω cm.

To clarify the units of the cell's resistivities and capacitance, we will calculate the values of the components of the four-element model of a cell (figure 2.4(*a*)). We will assume that the cell is cubic and has the dimensions of 10 μm × 10 μm × 10 μm and is surrounded by a 100 μm film of extracellular fluid with a resistivity of 100 Ω cm. Since the sides of the cube are in parallel with the surrounding fluid, we will ignore the resistance and capacitance of the membrane on the sides of the cube. The values of components are:

$$R_m = 100\ \Omega\ \mathrm{cm}^2/100\ \mu\mathrm{m}^2 = 100\ \mathrm{M}\Omega$$

$$C_m = 1\ \mu\mathrm{F/cm}^2 \times 100\ \mu\mathrm{m}^2 = 1 \times 10^{-18}\ \mathrm{F}$$

$$R_i = 60\ \Omega\ \mathrm{cm} \times 10\ \mu\mathrm{m}/100\ \mu\mathrm{m}^2 = 60\ \mathrm{k}\Omega$$

$$R_e = 100\ \Omega\ \mathrm{cm} \times 10\ \mu\mathrm{m}/(10\ \mu\mathrm{m} \times 100\ \mu\mathrm{m} \times 4) = 2500\ \Omega.$$

2.4 FREQUENCY DEPENDENCE OF TISSUE IMPEDANCE

The impedance of tissues decreases slowly with an increase in frequency. This behavior is related to the cellular structure of tissues and the frequency dependence of the membrane characteristics. The frequency dependence can be separated into three main regions. These regions are caused by the three dispersions (changes in magnitude) observed in the permittivity (ε) variations with frequency and are labeled α, β and γ (figure 2.6). The α dispersion decreases ε between 10 Hz and 10 kHz and is caused by interfacial polarizations and surface ionic conduction at membrane boundaries. The β dispersion decreases ε between 100 kHz and 10 MHz and is caused by the membrane capacitance short circuiting the membrane resistance. The γ dispersion is in the microwave frequency range (1 to 100 GHz) and is caused by the relaxation of the water molecules in the intracellular fluid (Pethig 1979).

The decrease in impedance varies between tissues and some tissues do not experience major variations. Zheng *et al* (1984) showed that the longitudinal impedance of skeletal muscle did not vary in the frequency range from 1 Hz to 1 MHz while the transverse impedance decreased to 0.1 of the low-frequency impedance.

If we apply a sinusoidal voltage V to a tissue with an admittance $Y = G + j\omega C$, two current types flow, a conduction current ($I_c = VG$) and a displacement current ($I_d = CdV/dt = V2\pi fC$). Figure 2.9 shows the variations of I_c and I_d with frequency for soft tissue. For frequencies lower than 100 kHz, the conduction current is much higher than the displacement current and the impedance of tissues is mainly resistive.

Figures 2.2, 2.10, 2.11 and 2.12 show examples of the frequency dependence of tissue impedance and are described elsewhere in this chapter.

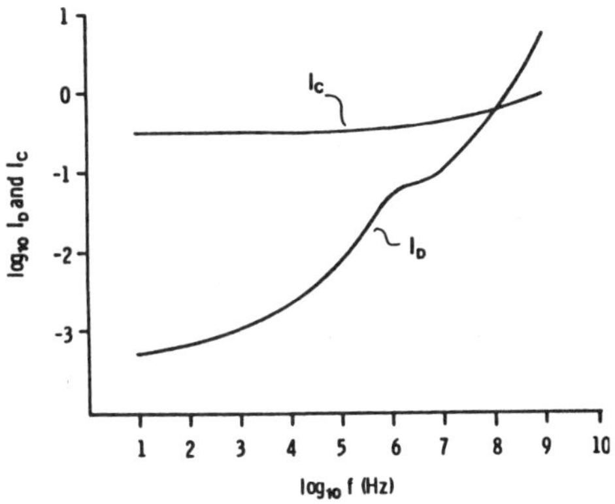

Figure 2.9 The conduction current I_c is much greater than the displacement current I_d at frequencies used for impedance imaging (Brown 1983).

2.5 TEMPERATURE DEPENDENCE OF TISSUE IMPEDANCE

Tissue impedance decreases with an increase in temperature. This dependence, however, varies with the applied frequency and the water content of the tissue. Pethig (1979) cited values for the change in tissue resistivity of $\Delta\rho/\rho = -1\%/^\circ C$ and permittivity of $\Delta\varepsilon/\varepsilon = +1.2\%/^\circ C$ at 1 MHz. Zheng *et al* (1984) measured the temperature dependence of the total impedance of skeletal muscle between 5°C and 40°C and found that the impedance changes by –2%/°C. Schwan (1957) provided detailed information about the temperature dependence of the resistivity and permittivity in the ultrahigh-frequency range (50–900 MHz). This phenomenon suggests that we can monitor tissues during hyperthermia treatment by monitoring the changes in their resistivities.

2.6 TEMPORAL DEPENDENCE

The impedance of some tissues varies with time because of the continuous change in the structure of the tissue. The change in the structure can be a change in the volume, flow, or concentration of elements in tissues. The lung is an example of tissue that changes in volume. Barber and Brown (1984) reported that the impedance of canine lung varied between 727 Ω cm at expiration to 2363 Ω cm at inhalation.

The blood in tissues is an example of the flow and concentration variation in the tissue. Hill and Thompson (1975) studied the dependence of blood resistivity on the hematocrit (Hct), which is the percentage of blood cells in blood, and developed a formula for the resistivity of blood:

$$\rho = 2.102\text{Hct} + 30.098\ (\Omega\ \text{cm}). \tag{2.11}$$

Barber and Brown (1984) noted that the resistance of the blood varies with the velocity of the blood by up to 14%.

Another important example of the temporal dependence of tissue impedance is the degradation of tissue after death. The change of the electrical characteristics of tissue after death could be related to the breakdown in the cellular membrane properties. Schwan (1957) provided detailed information on the change in the impedance of muscle tissues after excision and noted that this dependence is more apparent in the α frequency range and less apparent at higher frequencies. Zheng *et al* (1984) noted variations in the transverse impedance of skeletal muscle tissue of up to 20% increase and down to 70% decrease one hour after excision.

2.7 ANISOTROPIC DEPENDENCE OF TISSUE IMPEDANCE

Some tissues, such as those of bone and skeletal muscle, have a definite geometrical structure which causes an anisotropic dependence of tissue impedance. Burger and Dongen (1961) developed an equation for the conductivity of anisotropic tissue at an angle ϕ to the parallel direction of the tissue:

$$\sigma(\phi) = (\sigma_{\parallel}{}^2\cos^2\phi + \sigma_{\perp}{}^2\sin^2\phi)^{1/2} \tag{2.12}$$

where $\sigma(\phi)$ is the conductivity at angle ϕ, $\sigma_{\parallel}$ is the conductivity in the parallel direction and $\sigma_{\perp}$ is the conductivity in the perpendicular direction.

Figure 2.10 shows the impedance of bone in the axial, radial and circumferential directions (Reddy and Saha 1984). Figure 2.11 shows the Cole–Cole plots for the transverse and longitudinal skeletal muscle impedance (Epstein and Foster 1983). The transverse impedance was ten times the longitudinal impedance at low frequencies.

2.8 SKIN IMPEDANCE

The skin consists mainly of the stratum corneum which is composed of layers of dead cells (keratin layers) of total thickness of about 40 μm (Yamamoto and Yamamoto 1976a). Rosell *et al* (1988a) studied the impedance of unabraded skin and found that skin impedance for 1 cm^2 can be as high as 1 MΩ at low frequencies (figure 2.2). Yamamoto and Yamamoto (1976a, b) studied the decrease of skin impedance during skin stripping. They removed the stratum corneum by step-wise stripping using cellulose tape. Figure 2.12 shows that the outermost layers have the highest impedance and that the impedance drops by more than 50% after the first stage of stripping.

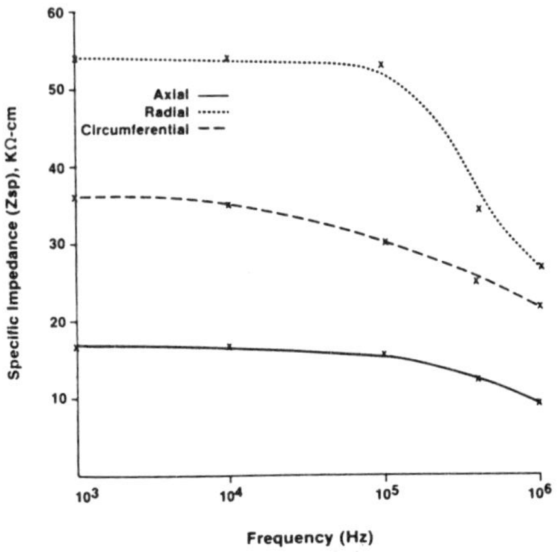

Figure 2.10 The specific impedance of bone tissue decreases with frequency (Reddy and Saha 1984).

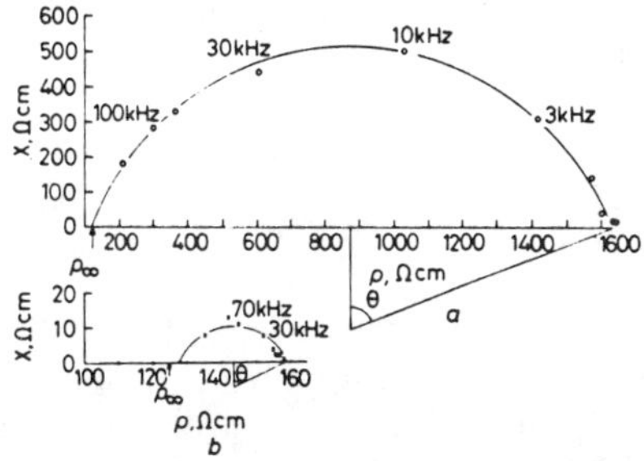

Figure 2.11 Cole–Cole plots for the transverse (a) and longitudinal (b) impedance of skeletal muscles (Epstein and Foster 1983).

We can model the skin with a three-element circuit as shown in figure 2.4(b). Pethig (1984) reported the following values for the components of the skin model: $C = 4.6$ nF/cm^2, $R_2 = 34.9$ kΩ cm^2 and $R_1 = 6.2$ kΩ cm^2. Note that the values are reported per unit area because the skin has a constant thickness of 40 μm.

The high and variable impedance of skin, especially at low frequencies for unabraded skin, suggests that biopotential amplifiers should have a very high input impedance to avoid the conversion of the common-mode voltage to differential voltage.

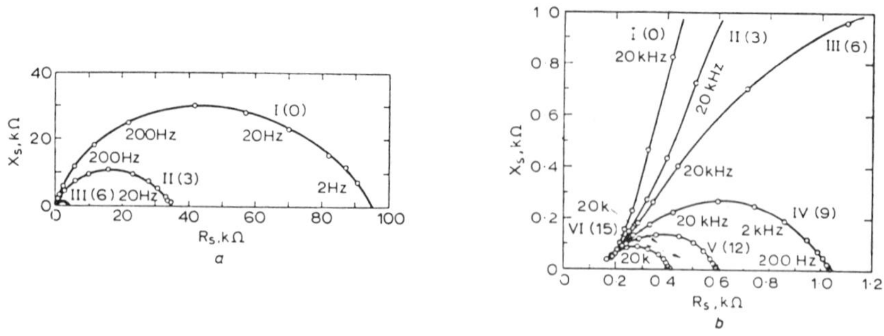

Figure 2.12 The impedance of the skin decreases with the removal of the stratum corneum (the number in parentheses shows the number of strippings) (Yamamoto and Yamamoto 1976a).

2.9 ORGAN IMPEDANCE

Figure 2.13 shows mammalian organ impedances from 20 to 100 kHz (Barber and Brown 1984, Rush *et al* 1963, Schwan and Kay 1956). Other good reviews of organ impedances are by Geddes and Baker (1967) and more recently by Stuchly and Stuchly (1984).

2.10 PHANTOMS

A phantom is a box of rectangular or cylindrical shape that is filled with materials of homogenous resistivity or with a collection of separate materials of different resistivities. Phantoms provide controllable mediums that can be used for the calibration and testing of systems that measure tissue impedance such as EIT systems. Figure 2.14 shows the phantom that was used by Sakamoto *et al* (1987).

The materials used inside the phantoms are commonly of water, agar and other substances such as NaCl and polyvinyl chloride (PVC). When all of those components are boiled together, a gelatinous substance of reasonable strength results that can be molded into different shapes or stored for later use. Yorkey (1986) used 1.5 g of agar powder to 100 ml of distilled water and added (m) g of NaCl. He calculated the conductivity of the substance from:

$$\sigma = 0.02m \quad (\mathrm{S/cm}). \tag{2.13}$$

For salt or distilled water with NaCl only, he calculated the conductivity from:

$$\sigma = 0.04m \quad (\mathrm{S/cm}). \tag{2.14}$$

Tissue	Resistivity
Cerebrospinal fluid	65 Ω cm
Plasma	66 Ω cm
Blood	150 Ω cm
Liver	350 Ω cm 550 Ω cm
Human arm	240 Ω cm (longitudinal) 675 Ω cm (transverse)
Skeletal muscle	125 Ω cm (longitudinal) 1800 Ω cm (transverse) 150 Ω cm (longitudinal) 2300 Ω cm (transverse) 530 Ω cm (average of above)
Cardiac muscle	160 Ω cm (longitudinal) 424 Ω cm (transverse) 575 Ω cm (longitudinal) 5181 Ω cm (transverse) 410 ~ 750 Ω cm (average values)
Neural tissue –gray matter –white matter	580 Ω cm 284 Ω cm 682 Ω cm
Lung	727 ~ 2363 Ω cm 2100 ± 17% Ω cm 1120 Ω cm 1275 Ω cm
Fat	2060 Ω cm 2500 Ω cm 2720 Ω cm
Bone	16600 Ω cm

Figure 2.13 The resistivity of organ tissue at low frequencies (20 to 100 kHz) (Barber and Brown 1984).

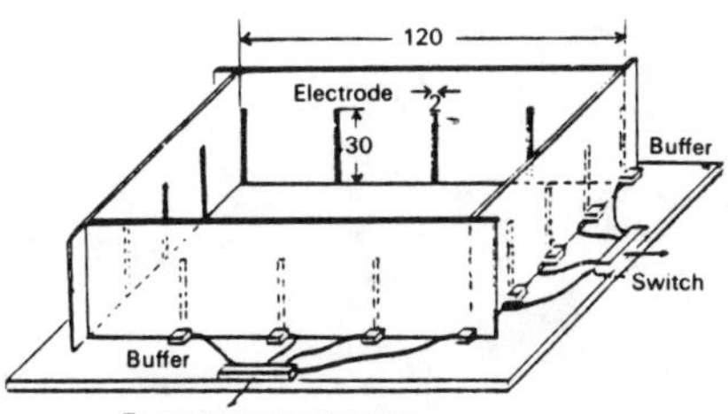

Figure 2.14 A 16–electrode physical phantom made of printed circuit boards (Sakamoto *et al* 1987).

Kato and Ishida (1987) developed equations (2.15) and (2.16) below for a phantom material that was constructed from water, agar powder, sodium azide (NaN_3) and PVC and was used in the frequency range 5–40 MHz. In a different paper, Kato *et al* (1986) provided the equations for materials constructed from water, agar powder, sodium azide and NaCl:

$$\sigma = 4.144 \times 10^{-3}(146.6N + 0.059)(85 - P)^{1.235} \text{ (S/m)} \tag{2.15}$$

$$\varepsilon = 79.25 - 1.009P \tag{2.16}$$

where N is the ratio (weight of NaN_3/weight of water) and was varied between 0 and 8×10^{-3}. P is {weight of PVC/(weight of PVC + weight of water)} × 100 and was varied between 0 and 44.4. The agar powder concentration ({weight of agar powder/(weight of agar powder + weight of water)} × 100) was fixed at 4%.

One disadvantage in using phantoms is the lack of a parallel component to the skin impedance. This can cause errors especially for two-electrode measurement systems.

2.11 STUDY QUESTIONS

2.1 Define, give units for, and give equations that relate impedance, conductivity σ and dielectric constant ε.
2.2 Give the equation for the impedance Z, as a function of frequency ω, and variables from question 2.1.
2.3 Sketch a plot of σ and ε as a function of frequency from 1 Hz to 1 MHz. Indicate the relative contribution of each to Z on the same plot.
2.4 List σ for the ten most important organs.
2.5 Explain on a cellular basis why ε varies with frequency.
2.6 Sketch a typical variation of tissue impedance of an internal organ with frequency.
2.7 Fit a three-element model to the sketch in the previous question.
2.8 Sketch a Cole–Cole plot for question 2.7, label all important parameters and explain how we can use it.
2.9 Repeat the previous three questions for skin.

3

Electrodes

John G Webster

An electrode is a transducer that converts the electronic current in a wire to an ionic current in an electrolyte, such as tissue. Contact impedance between the electrode and the tissue must be small and known in order to design instruments and reconstruct impedance images. We must use electrodes of reasonable materials and size to interface between the metal of the instrument and the ionic conductors in the tissue. There are a number of engineering tradeoffs we will consider to select optimal electrodes.

3.1 MATERIALS

3.1.1 Metals

Most electrodes are made of metal. It is easy to connect the metal wires from an instrument to the metal of a plate electrode. The electrode is placed on the skin and normally a viscous saline gel is added to improve contact between the metal and the skin. At the interface between the metal and the electrolyte, a chemical reaction must take place in order for current to flow. Electrodes are frequently coated with salts that facilitate this chemical reaction and this lowers the impedance. For example, silver is frequently coated with silver chloride to achieve the very reversible reaction, $AgCl + e^- = Ag + Cl^-$. Thus charges in the form of electrons in the metal convert the AgCl to Ag and yield ionic flow in the electrolyte as Cl^-. When easy reactions such as this are not available, more difficult reactions will occur, such as the electrolysis of water. These require higher voltage, which results in higher impedance, and also the formation of gas bubbles, which changes the electrode area. It is possible that metal ions driven electrophoretically into the body could cause toxic irritation.

Silver electrodes coated with silver chloride are the most common used for measuring the ECG. Tin/tin-chloride is also used. Stainless steel is a common electrode material as it does not corrode. Noble metals such as gold and platinum are used in specialized applications.

3.1.2 Carbon

Carbon is frequently added to plastic materials to make them conductive. For example silicone rubber is normally an insulator. When graphite powder is added before polymerization, resistivity can be lowered to 8 Ω cm. Metal can form a back plate for the conductive rubber, but frequently metal pins are inserted into cylindrical holes in the rubber to make a press-fit connection. Carbon electrodes cannot introduce any toxic products into the body, as some metal electrodes can. Carbon electrodes are also radiotransparent, which yields better X-ray pictures.

3.1.3 Adhesive polymers

Karaya gum is a natural polymer. Adding NaCl and other chemicals yields a conductive adhesive polymer (Carim 1988). The principal advantage of these metal-backed electrodes is that they perform a combined function of pressure-sensitive tape and gel and thus are compact. Their impedance is satisfactory for use as ECG electrodes, but is high for use in imaging.

Synthetic polymers are also used in electrodes. Polyvinyl pyrrolidone is a hydrophilic, elastomeric, water-insoluble pressure-sensitive adhesive. Polymerized acrylic acid is a nonirritating, conformable, cohesive, hydrophilic polymer. Like karaya gum, these have been used as ECG electrodes, but also have high impedance.

3.1.4 Electrolytes

Metal and conductive rubber electrodes can be placed directly on the skin. The electrode to skin impedance will be high at first, but within a minute or so perspiration hydrates the skin and the impedance decreases to a reasonable value. However, many applications use a conductive gel between the metal and the skin to promote uniform contact, and supply a large excess of moisture to fully hydrate the skin. This supplies a more concentrated electrolyte than that supplied by perspiration and this diffuses into the skin and lowers the skin impedance.

The electrolyte in the body is about 0.9% NaCl. Thus this would be an ideal electrolyte to put on the surface of the body to avoid irritation. To achieve lower impedance, 4% NaCl is used, which approximates the concentration of salt water in the sea. 20% NaCl is quite irritating, as anyone who has swum in Great Salt Lake or the Dead Sea can testify. 4% NaCl is placed in a thickening gel and antibacterial agents added. The resulting gel is messy, but effective in lowering contact impedance.

If using a gel on the skin, we must ensure that body movement will not smear the gel under one electrode so that it makes contact with the gel under an adjacent electrode. This would provide a short circuit between electrodes outside the relatively high impedance of the skin.

3.1.5 Adhesives

There must be a means for holding the electrode on the body. For measuring the diagnostic ECG in a resting subject, rubber straps encircle the limbs and chest to hold reusable plate electrodes in place. For impedance imaging, an elastic strap or girdle may be similarly useful. For monitoring the ECG in a moving subject, disposable pressure-sensitive electrodes are used. These have an adhesive ring around the central electrode. The pressure-sensitive adhesive must have sufficient tack to hold on, yet not be so aggressive that it removes skin when removed. The adhesive material must not irritate the skin.

3.2 IMPEDANCE VERSUS FREQUENCY

Figure 3.1 shows that the impedance of a pair of metal electrodes separated by paper towel saturated with electrode gel decreases with frequency. Note that for materials such as zinc, carbon and German silver, the impedance is low. When extrapolated to the usual frequencies for impedance imaging of 12–100 kHz, impedances would be 10 Ω or less. For other materials such as nickel and tin, the impedance is high, and might cause problems for impedance imaging. Some workers have used Ag/AgCl or similar low-impedance electrodes to construct impedance imaging physical phantoms. The results may be somewhat misleading because they do not include the effects of the skin impedance, which is in series with the electrode contact impedance. Figure 2.2 shows that the skin impedance at 12 kHz is about 1000 Ω cm^2 and that at 100 kHz is about 200 Ω cm^2. Compared to this, the impedance of the electrode is negligible and a realistic phantom would have electrodes that simulate the skin—perhaps by adding a layer of dielectric material such as thin plastic or cellophane over the electrodes. This is difficult to do because to obtain the capacitive 200 Ω, the thickness would have to be

$$t = X_C \omega \varepsilon_0 \varepsilon_r A = (200\ \Omega)(2\pi 100\ \text{kHz})(8.8 \times 10^{-12}\ \text{F/m})(3)(0.01\ \text{m})^2 = 0.33\ \mu\text{m}$$

where ε_0 is the dielectric constant for vacuum, ε_r is the relative dielectric constant of plastic, and A is the area. This small thickness suggests that the capacitance of the skin is formed by few layers of flattened cells in the barrier layer. It would be difficult to achieve such a thin layer of plastic because most plastics are made only as thin as 380 μm (1.5 mil). A possibility would be to use polyimide, which can be made in layers 1 μm thick or to anodize a metal such as aluminum in a manner similar to making an electrolytic capacitor.

Note that the shapes of the curves of figure 3.1 are similar to those of figure 2.2 and figure 2.10—the impedance in both decreases with frequency. Thus we can use the same three-element model and Cole–Cole plot to characterize electrode impedance as we did for skin impedance.

3.3 SIZE AND GEOMETRIES

3.3.1 Area

The conductance of an electrode increases linearly with area. Thus we would give the conductance of an electrode in units of siemens per square centimeter (S cm^{-2}). When we multiply by increasing electrode area, conductance

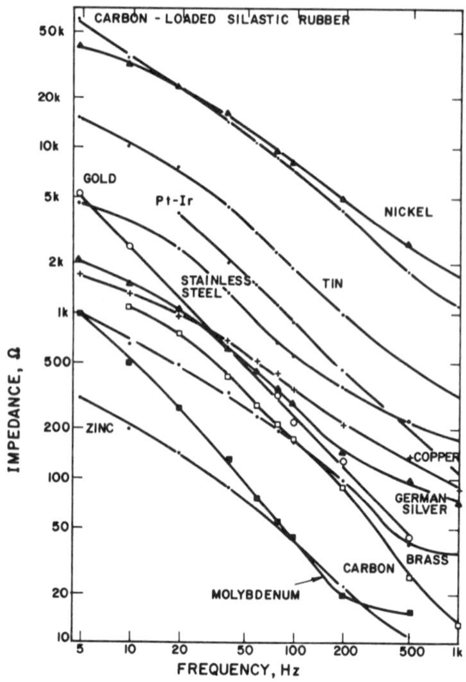

Figure 3.1 The impedance of a pair of 1 cm^2 electrodes decreases with frequency. Impedance of Ag/AgCl electrodes is less than 10 Ω for these frequencies (Das and Webster 1980).

increases and we end up with units of siemens. Similarly the impedance of an electrode is equal to the reciprocal of the conductance or S^{-1} cm^2, or Ω cm^2. In this case, when we divide by increasing electrode area, impedance decreases and we end up with units of ohms.

Figure 3.2(*a*) shows the easiest way to measure electrode impedances—by placing them face to face. But figure 3.2(*b*) shows that isolated electrodes have nonuniform current densities. At the edges, the current density is very high and in the center, much lower (Wiley and Webster 1982). To measure the electrode impedance, we must place a voltage-measuring electrode very near the measured electrode. We will always include some tissue impedance and thus can only measure the approximate electrode impedance. At low frequencies, the high skin impedance makes the current density uniform. But at high frequencies, the high resistance of the skin is short circuited by its capacitance and we obtain the situation shown in figure 3.2(*b*).

3.3.2 Geometry

Yorkey *et al* (1985) found electrode contact impedances of 70 Ω and electronic switch impedances of 130 Ω. These created such large errors in their physical phantom that they developed the driven electrode system shown in figure 3.3.

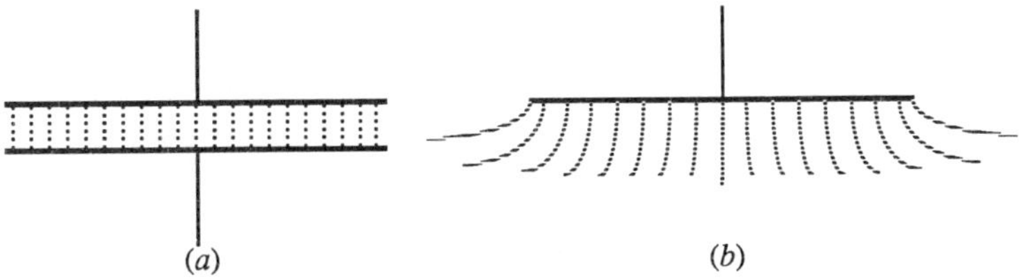

Figure 3.2 (*a*) Electrode impedances measured face-to-face assume that the current density is uniform. (*b*) Electrode impedance from an isolated electrode yields measurements for nonuniform current density.

Measuring voltage on an electrode different from the current electrode minimizes the effect of contact impedance. However, the large current electrodes along the side provided a low-impedance shunt pathway for the current that did not exist in the center and distorted the current density. They solved this problem by making very narrow electrodes that had a small circumferential dimension.

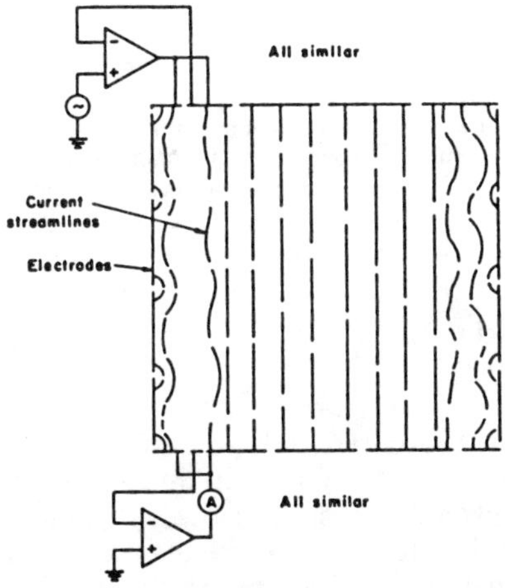

Figure 3.3 The driven electrode system measures the voltage at the center electrode and drives current though the annular ring electrode around it. However, vertical currents were shunted by the large side electrodes and distorted the current density (Yorkey *et al* 1985).

3.4 TWO VERSUS FOUR ELECTRODES

Figure 3.4 shows that a two-electrode system measures electrode contact impedance plus tissue impedance. Yorkey *et al* (1985) had problems with a two-electrode system and achieved improvement by changing to a four-electrode driven system. Barber *et al* (1983) used a four-electrode system in which they introduced current on two neighboring electrodes and measured voltages on all other electrodes. Gisser *et al* (1987) measured voltage on the same electrodes that carry current and thus it would seem that this is a two-electrode system. They argue however that they really have a 32-electrode system, and because they introduce current on all electrodes, they achieve the same current profiles under the skin that they do outside the skin because the current lines are approximately parallel for their $\cos\theta$ current distribution.

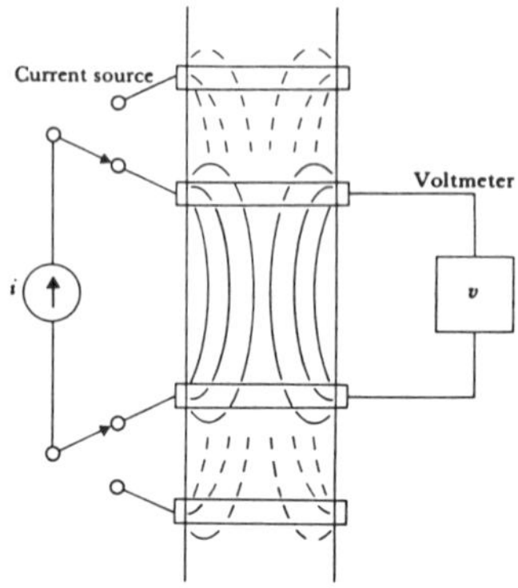

Figure 3.4 In a two-electrode system, switches are in the position shown, so the voltmeter measures tissue impedance plus electrode contact impedance. In a four-electrode system, switches are thrown to the other position and the voltmeter does not measure electrode contact impedance (Webster 1978b).

3.5 GUARD ELECTRODE

Figure 3.5 shows that a guard electrode is useful in focussing the measured current into a region of interest. Henderson and Webster (1978) used a guard electrode in their two-electrode system. However, Plonsey and Collin (1977) concluded that a guarded system has no advantages over an unguarded system. Use of a guard in impedance imaging is probably not useful because the current supplied by the guarding electrode is not measured, and would distort current density in the region of interest.

3.6 ELECTRODE APPLICATIONS

3.6.1 Electrodes on humans

Henderson and Webster (1978) made their 144 electrodes from 15-mm-diameter coat snaps fastened through rubber bed sheeting. At 100 kHz their impedance was much smaller than the skin impedance.

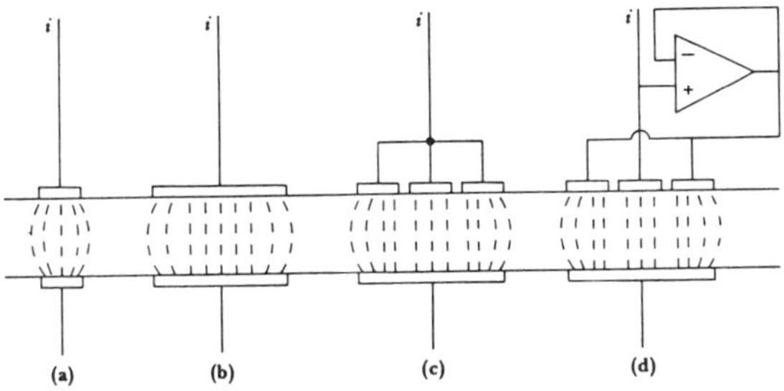

Figure 3.5 (*a*) Small electrodes have considerable fringing, so they emphasize impedance changes in the high-current density region near electrodes. (*b*) Large electrodes produce a more uniform current density. (*c*) Splitting the electrode into a center electrode plus an annular guard electrode does not change current distribution. (*d*) Driving the guard with a unity-gain follower causes current *i* to flow only through the central region (Webster 1978b).

Barber *et al* (1983) apply 16 disposable ECG electrodes at equal distances around the chest. At 50 kHz their impedance was much smaller than the skin impedance. Their four-electrode system is insensitive to electrode/skin contact impedance.

Isaacson showed a videotape in his talk "Problems in adaptive current tomography" at the Duke–North Carolina NSF/ERC Workshop, "Impedance-based cardiovascular measurements" April 4, 1989. In it he wore rectangular conductive adhesive electrodes with the long dimension vertical, that filled most of the circumference of his chest, to image resistivity changes during ventilation. To lower skin impedance, he stripped the outer layer of the skin by applying masking tape, then stripping it off.

3.6.2 Electrodes in physical phantoms

Yorkey *et al* (1985) constructed a physical phantom from printed circuit board glass-epoxy with the copper-etched electrodes overcoated with tin. This made their four-electrode driven electrode system easy to construct. The electrodes were 30 mm on a side and measured 20 Ω at 100 kHz.

Kim *et al* (1987) constructed a physical phantom using Ag/AgCl electrodes. When each of the 32 electrodes was placed in series with a 100 Ω resistor, the standard deviation of the current variation was 0.148%.

Gisser *et al* (1987) constructed a physical phantom using 30 × 40 mm Pt/Ir electrodes and achieved 5 Ω impedance at 12 kHz. The electrodes were spaced 1 mm apart and thus filled almost all the available space.

No one yet has built a phantom that simulates the impedance of the skin, as noted in Section 3.2.

3.6.3 Future electrodes

For dynamic measurements, measuring and applying 16 disposable ECG electrodes is a time-consuming chore. Applying a stretchable belt with reusable electrodes already in it should be more convenient and less expensive. It should be of a washable material such as spandex. Initial attempts have encountered the problem that electrodes at the concavities of the thorax at the front and rear midlines do not make contact on some persons..

For static measurements, the electrode positions must be fixed. Thus they must be in a rigid line or circle. Applying a rigid line of electrodes to one side of the tissue seems reasonable. Applying a rigid circle around the thorax would make breathing difficult and lying down unpleasant for subjects, even if it were a hinged clamshell. The space between the circle and the thorax would have to be filled with gelatinous conducting material or else the body would have to be immersed in a tank of saline.

If low spatial resolution is acceptable, a stretchable girdle containing electrodes might yield some useful information such as breathing rate or volume. Rather than constraining the electrodes to a single plane, more information might be obtained by spreading the electrodes in a polkadotted array all over the thorax.

Pilkington *et al* (1989) suggested the utilization of an esophageal reference electrode to enhance impedance imaging. They showed the result of an analysis of the expected improvement in distinguishability (see Section 12.4) of target inhomogeneities when an esophageal reference electrode was located on the target-body interface. Their analysis showed that there is an enhancement in target distinguishability of approximately two for the one-dimensional, two-dimensional (for large radius target) and three-dimensional (for large radius target) cases. However, for small diameter targets of radius < 0.1 in the two-dimensional and three-dimensional cases, the enhancement increase is considerable (>6 in the two-dimensional and >30 in the three-dimensional cases) probably due to the focusing of static current fields on the small target near the esophageal electrode. However, the usefulness of the esophageal reference electrode in EIT needs more research.

3.7 STUDY QUESTIONS

3.1 Give the units for measuring conductance and impedance per unit area.

3.2 Sketch the skin impedance and stainless steel electrode impedance vs. frequency on a common plot from 1 Hz to 1 MHz.

3.3 Calculate the best-fit three-element models for the skin and electrode impedance in the previous question.

3.4 Estimate the impedance for a 1 cm^2 skin/electrode combination at 50 kHz. Estimate the error this would cause in a two-electrode circuit compared to a four-electrode circuit.

3.5 Sketch the current lines under a normal electrode and under a guarded electrode.

4

Current Generators

Daniel J Nowicki

To measure an unknown impedance, we must do one of two things. Either we must apply a known voltage across the object and then measure the current through it, or we must inject a known current into that object and measure the voltage across it. Both of these methods have been used for various EIT and similar systems. In this chapter we will discuss ways of implementing the method of current injection, particularly those being developed at the University of Wisconsin–Madison in its 50 kHz, 32-electrode current injection system.

4.1 INTRODUCTION

Impedance imaging systems have included a 144-electrode impedance camera using voltage input (Henderson and Webster 1978), a 192-electrode voltage input system (Kim and Woo 1987), a 16-electrode EIT system with one current generator (Brown and Seagar 1987), a 32-current generator EIT system (Newell *et al* 1988) and a one-generator banded electrode impedance measuring system (Goovaerts *et al* 1988).

This chapter will include possible oscillators and voltage-controlled current sources. We will then discuss in Chapter 5 different means of amplifying and demodulating the signal to measure the voltage response.

4.2 CURRENT INPUT VERSUS VOLTAGE INPUT

In a system where we are measuring some electrical parameter from a patient, an unknown contact impedance exists between the electrode and the patient's tissue. As stated in Chapter 3, a four-electrode system helps to reduce the problems with contact impedance experienced by two-electrode systems.

Still, in a four-electrode system, contact impedance can be a factor affecting system accuracy. Later in the chapter we show that a good current source has high output impedance, while a good voltage source has low output impedance. This means that while the contact impedance will be negligible for a current source, it will degrade the operation of a voltage source. Likewise, the input impedance of a voltmeter is high, while the input impedance of an ammeter should be near zero. Hence the contact impedance will be much smaller than a voltmeter's input impedance, but will be large compared with an ammeter's input impedance. This suggests that a system using current injection and voltage measurement would produce the best results with an unknown, varying contact impedance.

The current injection method does require more complex hardware than a system using voltage application and current measurement. But, because it is more accurate, at present most groups active in EIT research use current injection; this will therefore be the method that we shall discuss.

4.3 SYSTEM OVERVIEW

The hardware for an electrical impedance tomograph has many components, each of which requires special consideration and design.

Figure 4.1 shows a hardware block diagram for an electrical impedance tomograph. On the right is the computer control port. Commands are sent through this port to configure the device. The digital commands are decoded and sent to the current sources, switching network and variable-gain amplifier. An oscillator provides the carrier signal to both the current sources and the demodulator. After the currents are injected into the patient, a switching network chooses the measurement locations. The amplified signal is then demodulated to low frequencies so that it can be converted into digital form for the computer.

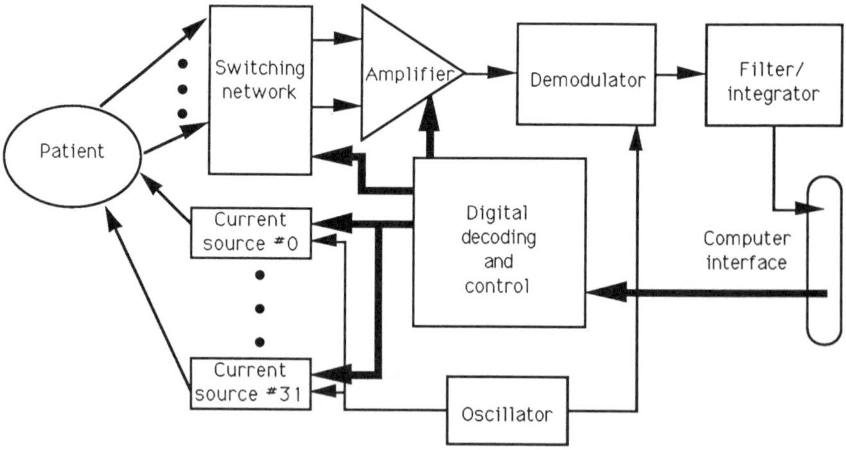

Figure 4.1 The hardware block diagram for a general electrical impedance tomograph. Bold lines indicate digital control.

4.4 OSCILLATORS

The master oscillator serves as a frequency and amplitude reference for all of the current source channels. As discussed in Chapter 5, the oscillator output may also serve as the switching function input for the demodulator. Most oscillators depart from our idealized requirements in two aspects: the output amplitude may vary over time, or it may contain some distortion from a pure sine wave.

As with all the other system components, the noise contribution from the oscillator depends on the demodulation technique employed. In Chapter 5 we give a detailed description of this noise contribution for the most typically used demodulator types, namely the multiplying and switching demodulators. In this section we will summarize those results as they apply to oscillator noise.

The output amplitude's time variation may not be a problem at all if it changes sufficiently slowly that a complete set of measurements can be taken before the amplitude varies by δ. (Here and throughout the text, δ represents the system's error tolerance. For 12-bit accuracy, $\delta = 1/4096$.) For a 32-electrode system with a conversion time of 300 μs per measurement, the amplitude must be stable for almost 10 ms. As discussed in Chapter 8, though, some data collection methods require multiple measurement sets for a number of current injection patterns. These methods will require even longer periods of amplitude stability.

If the amplitude does change during this time, some of the voltage measurements in the set will be inaccurate or, in other words, noisy. For an amplitude noise of ε, an oscillator amplitude of A and a system gain G, from equations (5.8) and (5.9), we can find the demodulator output. These equations are

$$|V_O V_M| \approx A^2 G(1 + 2\varepsilon) \tag{4.1}$$

and

$$|V_S V_M| = AG(1 + \varepsilon) \tag{4.2}$$

for multiplying and switching demodulators respectively. From these results, we can see that the measured value is incorrect by about two times and one times the amplitude noise for the multiplying and switching demodulators respectively.

The second issue that we must consider is the oscillator's harmonic distortion. Again from Chapter 5 we summarize the noise contribution from the harmonic amplitude coefficients C_n where n is the harmonic number. From equations (5.11) and (5.13) we find this error to be

$$\sum_{n=2}^{\infty} C_n{}^2 \tag{4.3}$$

and

$$\sum_{n=3}^{\infty} \frac{C_n}{n} \quad n \text{ odd} \tag{4.4}$$

for multiplying and switching demodulators respectively.

Because C_n is generally small for a good oscillator, the result of equation (4.3) will be smaller than that of equation (4.4). Of course, this also depends a great deal on the distribution of the coefficients in n, particularly if they are dominantly even or odd.

Although knowing the individual frequency components will give us an exact number for their noise contribution, measuring these components can be difficult with common instruments. More often, the total harmonic distortion, THD, is measured and discussed in specification sheets. This measure of waveform purity is traditionally used by audio engineers (Evans and Towers 1980), and is defined as

$$\text{THD} = \left(\frac{\sum_{n=2}^{\infty} C_n^2}{\sum_{n=1}^{\infty} C_n^2} \right)^{1/2} \times 100\ \% \tag{4.5}$$

where C_n is again the amplitude coefficient of the nth harmonic.

Frequency stability is sometimes a concern when dealing with oscillators. In our situation, the stability is not critical, because although there is some frequency dependence in our instrumentation and the patient's impedance, the change due to frequency is negligible over a wide range.

Oscillator implementation could take on different forms. Those discussed below range from variations of circuits used 50 years ago to those which rely on high-speed digital electronics.

4.4.1 FET-stabilized Wien-bridge

A simple Wien-bridge oscillator is shown in figure 4.2. It uses two poles in the positive feedback path balanced by the gain in the negative feedback path to produce a stable sinusoidal oscillation (Tobey *et al* 1971). If the gain is balanced, the circuit will oscillate at a frequency of $1/[2\pi(R_1C_1R_2C_2)^{1/2}]$. But, if the negative feedback's gain varies from the balance point, the oscillation will either die out or diverge until the operational amplifier (op amp) is driven toward saturation. Because of this some form of automatic gain control is used. Originally an incandescent lamp was placed in the negative feedback. As the filament is heated from the current flowing through it, its resistance changes, thus changing the gain of the feedback.

Newell *et al* (1988) implemented a one op-amp, 15 kHz oscillator which used a FET for stabilization rather than a bulb. The output amplitude is sampled with a zener diode peak detector, and is smoothed to control the gate of the FET. The FET then acts as a variable resistance under control of the gate.

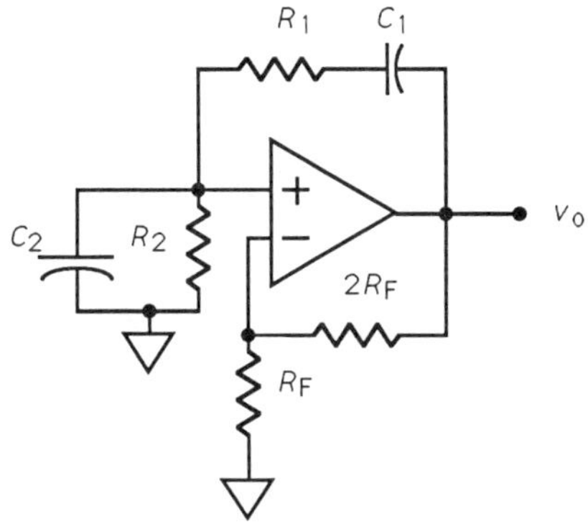

Figure 4.2 A simple one op-amp Wien-bridge oscillator. Frequency is determined by the components in the positive feedback. Amplitude is regulated and stable if the negative feedback ratio equals 1/3.

A three op-amp FET-stabilized Wien-bridge circuit is being used by the Wisconsin group. This version, shown in figure 4.3, is described in detail by Van der Walt (1981). The primary bridge consists of an oscillator, top left. The oscillator output is full-wave rectified and then compared to the reference voltage v_r. After filtering, this comparison signal is used to bias a FET which acts as a variable resistor in the negative feedback path for the oscillator.

Although Wien-bridge oscillators are quite old, their performance rivals any other oscillator in use. Van der Walt's 5 kHz oscillator had a distortion as low as 0.01% and the Wisconsin group 50 kHz oscillator has a distortion of 0.3%.

4.4.2 Monolithic function generators

Integrated circuit function generators such as the XR-2206 by Exar (EXAR Corporation 1987) can produce sine waves with less than 0.5% distortion. Because this distortion is mostly due to ripples at the signal peaks, it would most likely have a frequency three times the harmonic. With this distortion, it may cause errors for both multiplying and switching demodulators as shown by equations (4.3) and (4.4).

4.4.3 Digital function generation

Digitized waveforms may also be clocked out of a read-only memory (ROM) and then sent through a digital-to-analog converter (DAC). The output of the DAC is a staircase-like approximation to the desired waveform. For a generator that produces a function with many steps,the fundamental frequency component will be much larger than the frequencies that make up the steps. Thus the function may not have to be filtered if a phase-sensitive demodulator is used. Such a system is used by Brown and Seagar (1987) to produce a 51 kHz wave with 16 values per cycle from a 820 kHz clock. Rosell *et al* (1989) developed a parallel data acquisition system for EIT and they also used a digital signal generator. The injection current waveform was generated by digital synthesis with easy frequency selection among 10, 20, 40 and 80 kHz. They used phase shifting circuits to null out hardware-induced phase shifts for in-phase demodulation. The signal was transformer isolated and the power supply was made floating to allow the use of feedback to decrease the common mode voltage.

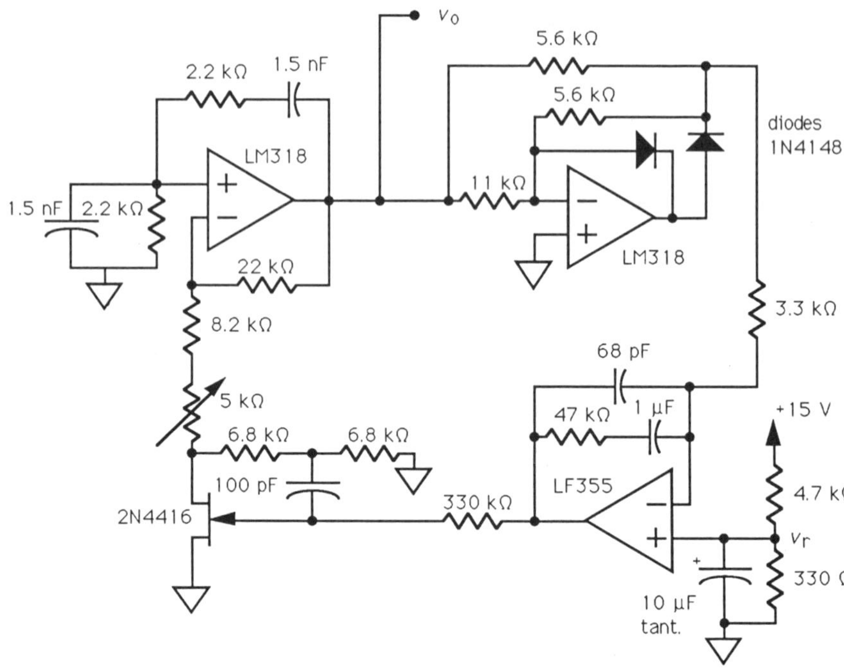

Figure 4.3 A three-op-amp Wien-bridge oscillator tuned for a 50 kHz output.

Evans and Towers (1980) give a detailed description of the distortion introduced for zero-order-hold and linear-interpolated waveform generators. A zero-order-hold (ZOH) generator simply outputs a constant value from a DAC for one sample period. The next sample will be a new value which is again held constant for the period. This gives the staircase look to a waveform generated in this way. A linear-interpolated, or first-order-hold (FOH), waveform is a closer approximation to the desired waveform. The time between each sample period is a smooth ramp, which will more closely follow the desired function if the sample period is chosen to be short enough. The output of each of these generators is shown in figure 4.4.

A sampled cosine wave with a frequency of ω_0 and sample period T can be expressed as

$$V_o(t) = \cos(\omega_0 t) \sum_{k=-\infty}^{\infty} \delta(t - kT).$$

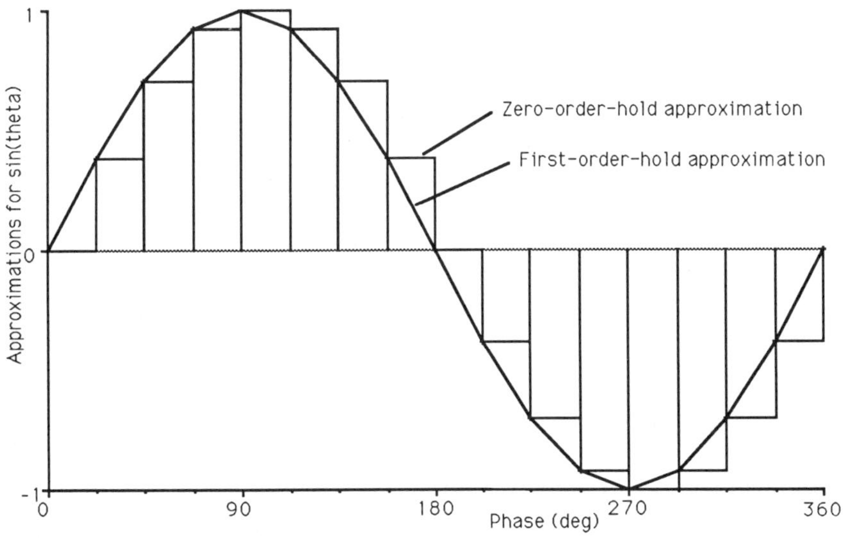

Figure 4.4 The sine approximation for zero-order-hold and first-order-hold digital oscillators with $N = 16$.

When this sampled waveform is output through a zero-order hold, the resulting waveform will have a spectrum with coefficients

$$|C_m| = \frac{1}{2}\left|\text{sinc}\left(\frac{m\pi}{N}\right)\right| \tag{4.6}$$

where m takes only those values determined by $f = (kN \pm 1)f_0 = mf_0$. For example if $N = 16$, m will take the values of 1, 15, 17, 31, 33, ... The coefficients for an interpolated wave will be

$$|C_m| = \frac{1}{2}\left|\text{sinc}\left(\frac{m\pi}{N}\right)\right|^2. \tag{4.7}$$

Because the sinc function never has an output greater than 1, the distortion coefficients of the first-order-hold waveform will always be less than those of the zero-order-hold waveform.

It is interesting to note that if we had chosen $N = 15$, the harmonics would be 1, 14, 16, 29, 31 etc. With a switching demodulator, where only the odd harmonics cause errors (equation (4.4)), the first significant harmonic would be at $n = 29$. This harmonic could easily be filtered with almost no phase or gain error introduced into the fundamental.

We can find the total harmonic distortion (THD) introduced by these two types of digital function generation from equations (4.8) and (4.9):

$$\mathrm{THD}_{\mathrm{ZOH}} = \left(1 - \left(\operatorname{sinc}\frac{\pi}{N}\right)^2\right)^{1/2} \times 100\% \tag{4.8}$$

$$\mathrm{THD}_{\mathrm{FOH}} = \left(1 - \frac{3 \times \left(\operatorname{sinc}\frac{\pi}{N}\right)^4}{2 + \cos\frac{2\pi}{N}}\right)^{1/2} \times 100\%. \tag{4.9}$$

From these equations, we find that the THD for a 32-sample-point waveform will be 5.665% for a ZOH and 0.144% for a FOH.

Towers (1982) describes a variety of hardware implementations for first-order-hold waveform generators.

4.5 VOLTAGE-CONTROLLED CURRENT SOURCES (VCCS)

Once we have produced the sine wave, we must convert it into a current whose magnitude is unaffected by load voltage. This load voltage is of course that presented by the subject's impedance to ground, Z_L. Figure 4.5 shows a model of a current source. For a perfect current source, output impedance Z_S will be infinite, and I_L will not vary with changes in Z_L.

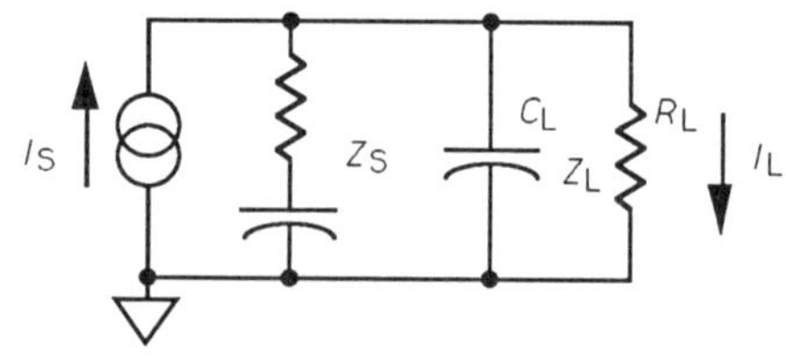

Figure 4.5 For an ideal current source, $R_S = \infty$ and I_L will not vary with changes in Z_L.

We would like to find the minimal value of Z_S so that the load current does not change significantly over the range of possible load impedances. This minimal value of Z_S is obtained by applying the current divider equation to figure 4.5 to obtain

$$I_L = I_S \frac{Z_S}{Z_S + Z_L} \ . \tag{4.10}$$

Equation (4.1) shows that two different load impedances, Z_1 and Z_2, will yield two different load currents, I_1 and I_2. We can simplify the equations produced by these two conditions to get

$$I_1 Z_S + I_1 Z_1 = I_S Z_S$$

$$I_2 Z_S + I_2 Z_2 = I_S Z_S.$$

These two equations for two unknowns can then be combined and reduced to

$$Z_S = \frac{I_2 Z_2 - I_1 Z_1}{I_1 - I_2} . \tag{4.11}$$

From this equation, we may calculate Z_S by substituting our maximal and minimal loads for Z_2 and Z_1 respectively. I_1 is the desired load current, and I_2 is the current that differs by at most a factor of δ from I_1. Over our range of interest for a real Z_L, 0 to 1 kΩ resistive, for 12 bit accuracy, if Z_S is purely resistive, it must be at least 4.7 MΩ.

As we will explain in Chapter 5, some demodulators are also sensitive to phase shift. Hence, for 12 bit accuracy, the current source output must change by less than 1.3°. Under these requirements, Z_S must be greater than 500 Ω – j44 kΩ.

Other requirements for our system include negligible direct-current (DC) output current, temporal stability and the ability to handle loads that include the series capacitance of the skin.

4.5.1 One op amp

The simplest version of a voltage-controlled current source (VCCS) is an inverting amplifier, with the load in the feedback path as shown in figure 4.6. For infinite op-amp gain, the inverting input of the op amp is a virtual ground. Because very little current enters the op amp at this input, the load current, I_L, is simply the input voltage divided by R_I. Of course, op-amp gain is not infinite, especially at the frequencies common to EIT, but for a typical open-loop gain of 600 at –90°, the output current error is less than 0.0003%. This is easily within acceptable limits. Even though this circuit is useful for some applications such as that described by Goovaerts *et al* (1988), it cannot be used for systems employing more than one current source, or systems with a grounded load.

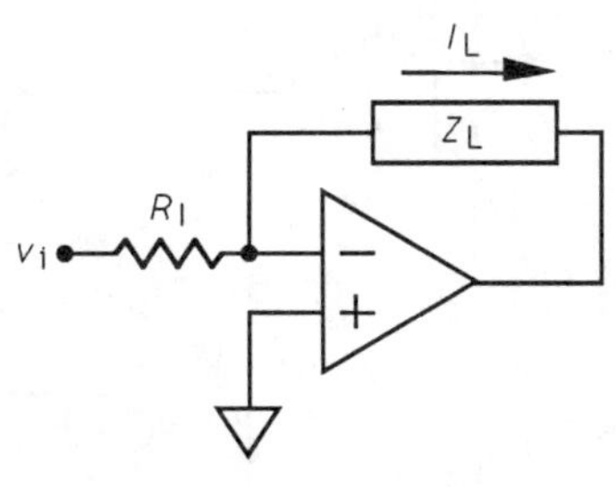

Figure 4.6 A simple one-op-amp VCCS requires that Z_L be floating.

4.5.2 One op amp, transformer-coupled

An extension of the above circuit DC-isolates the load from the op amp. In this way, the load can be grounded, and more than one current source can be used. This is accomplished by using a transformer to couple the load to the feedback path. Because the leakage inductance of the transformer lowers the output impedance, current sources of this type can only be used in systems that require lower accuracy, such as that described by Skidmore *et al* (1987).

4.5.3 Three op amp

Figure 4.7 shows a circuit used by Newell *et al* (1988) and first described in Wojslaw and Moustakas (1986). This circuit yields 12 bit accuracy at a frequency of 15 kHz. It also allows the use of grounded loads. v_l is inverted, to become v_f, and then added to v_i. The current through R_2 is then

$$I_2 = \frac{-(v_i + v_f) - v_l}{R_2} \tag{4.12}$$

or

$$I_2 = \frac{-v_i}{R_2} \quad \text{when } v_f = -v_l \tag{4.13}$$

assuming that the feedback path is ideal. If the buffer op amp is chosen to have high input impedance, all of current I_2 will flow through I_L.

At frequencies much higher than 15 kHz however, the phase shift introduced in the three-op-amp feedback path does not allow v_f to exactly equal $-v_l$. This means that equation (4.13) no longer holds true, unless components are added to compensate for the phase shift. It is therefore difficult to achieve high output impedances at high frequencies without adding further complexity to this circuit.

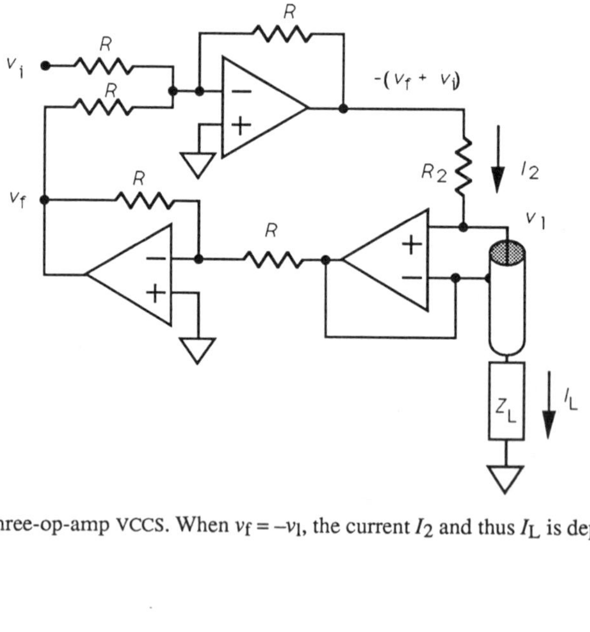

Figure 4.7 A three-op-amp VCCS. When $v_f = -v_l$, the current I_2 and thus I_L is dependent only on v_i.

4.5.4 One op amp with positive feedback

Figure 4.8 shows a circuit first described by Tobey *et al* (1971) being used by the Wisconsin group (Nowicki and Webster 1989). It achieves 12 bit accuracy at 50 kHz, and has the advantage of passing only enough DC current through the electrodes to bias the op amps. This minimizes polarization and corrosion which might occur if a sizable DC current passed through them for extended periods of time, as would happen in a constant monitoring situation.

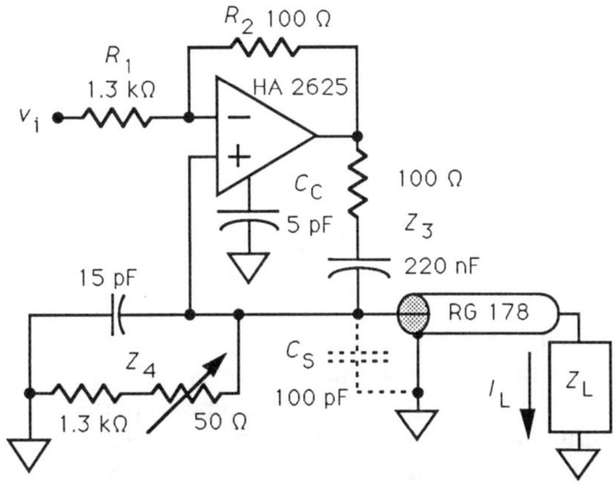

Figure 4.8 A one-op-amp with positive-feedback VCCS. For high output impedance, $R_1Z_3 = R_2Z_4$ where Z_3 and Z_4 are the total impedances.

Assuming an ideal op amp, the load current is given by

$$I_L = \frac{-v_i R_2 Z_4}{R_1 Z_3 Z_4 + Z_L(R_1 Z_3 - R_2 Z_4)} \tag{4.14}$$

or

$$I_L = \frac{-v_i}{Z_4} \quad \text{if } R_1 Z_3 = R_2 Z_4. \tag{4.15}$$

Although the op amp is not ideal, the gain and phase errors caused by it are small enough to be easily compensated by adjusting Z_4.

The DC blocking is accomplished by the capacitor at Z_3, while the capacitor at Z_4 is chosen to compensate for the phase shift introduced by Z_3.

The output impedance of a circuit of this type was found experimentally by varying the load resistance while measuring the voltage across a fixed, 39 Ω resistance in the load. For a load impedance from 39 to 1039 Ω, the voltage magnitude across the fixed resistor changed from 191.68 to 191.67 mV, or the current changed from 4.9149 to 4.9146 mA, while the phase changed by 0.22°. These results are then substituted into equation (4.11):

$$Z_S = \frac{(191.67\ @\ {-0.22°})\cdot 1039 - (191.68\ @\ 0°)\cdot 39}{(191.68\ @\ 0°) - (191.67\ @\ {-0.22°})} = 3.0\ \mathrm{k\Omega} - j260\ \mathrm{k\Omega}.$$

4.5.5 Current sources that use transistors

The op-amp current sources described above are easily implemented and will have a high output impedance as long as the frequency is within the range of the op amp. Some applications may require a higher frequency range, a larger load capability or reduced distortion. These applications may require the use of current sources that are either partially or wholly made of discrete transistors. King (1978) used a four transistor current source to minimize phase shifts for a device designed to operate between 10 and 100 kHz. Other sources use transistors within the feedback to boost current output, or current mirror combinations to boost output voltage swing.

4.5.6 Blocking DC currents from the VCCS

As discussed in Chapter 6, it is desirable to block any possible DC or low-frequency currents from passing through the patient. This can usually be achieved by placing a large capacitor, of a few microfarads, in series with the current source output.

If the capacitor is placed at the output, special attention must be paid to the current source's frequency response. At DC, general purpose op amps will have small offset currents and voltages. Usually these offsets will be unnoticed in an alternating-current (AC) system such as the one described here. However, these offsets will create the opportunity for a DC current to be produced by the VCCS, if it acts as a good current source at low frequencies. Also at DC, the blocking capacitor will present a near infinite load impedance. The small current through the large load will produce a voltage which will then drive the op amp towards saturation.

The low-frequency response of the VCCS can be lowered by using capacitive blocking in its positive feedback path. The capacitor in Z_3 accomplishes this blocking for the current source of figure 4.8.

4.6 OP AMPS

Because the open loop gain of an op amp decreases by 20 dB per decade at high frequencies, uncompensated op amps which generally have a wider bandwidth should be used in high-frequency circuits. For example, an op amp with a 2 MHz bandwidth will only have an open loop gain of 40 at 50 kHz, while a CA3100 with a 38 MHz bandwidth will have an open loop gain of about 1000 at this frequency. Of course, for low-gain configurations, the external compensation capacitances that are required will lower this gain. At 50 kHz, an HA2625 has an open loop gain of over 1500 with no compensation, but for a unity gain configuration where a 35 pF compensation is required, the open loop gain drops to about 300.

An op amp with finite gain G will have an output which is different from that determined by the ideal model. This difference is called the gain error. For a unity gain buffer whose real gain is $v_o/v_i \approx 1 - 1/G$, the gain error is $1/G$. If an op amp with gain of 300 were used, this error would be greater than 0.3%, which is unacceptable. Fortunately, at 50 kHz, the gain of an HA2625 is 300 with a phase shift of –90°. The gain error is therefore at about –90°, and will be filtered out if phase-sensitive demodulation is used.

Because the HA2625 also has high input impedance and low input bias current, it is being used by the Wisconsin group for most of the analog hardware in their electrical impedance tomograph.

4.7 DRIVEN SHIELD

To reduce crosstalk and to reduce interference pickup, the leads to the patient should be shielded in some way. The stray capacitance in the cables could add a shunt capacitance of 100 pF, if grounded shields were used. The shunt capacitance acts in much the same way as the output impedance of the VCCS, so we may model it by placing its parallel combination with Z_S into Z_S in equation (4.10). This means that, even if we attained an infinite output impedance from our current sources, for a load variation of 0 to 1 kΩ, the real component of the load current could vary by as much as 0.1%. Some method of avoiding this problem must be chosen.

If the shield is driven with approximately the same signal as the line, a much smaller current will flow through the cable's capacitance. This reduces the effective cable capacitance to as little as 1 pF. The shield may be driven either by an additional buffer or, as figure 4.7 shows, by one stage of the current source itself.

An alternative approach is to use the cable's capacitance as a circuit parameter in designing the current source, as is done for the VCCS in figure 4.8. If such a design is chosen, care should be practiced when changing the cable length.

4.8 SUMMARY

In this chapter we have discussed some of the components needed for the current injection half of the hardware. Several diverse implementations of function generators which could serve as the master oscillator have been discussed, along with the noise contribution of each. A few different op-amp-based voltage-controlled current sources have been presented.

4.9 STUDY QUESTIONS

4.1 What is the source of error in an impedance-measuring system that inputs voltage and measures current? Is there a similar problem for a system that inputs a current and measures voltage?

4.2 List the specifications on the oscillator amplitude function during one data-collection frame. Repeat for all iterations required for one image.
4.3 What disadvantage would a system using a square wave have?
4.4 Under what conditions of frequency, accuracy etc. would you choose each of the described oscillators?
4.5 List the advantages and disadvantages of each of the voltage-controlled current sources listed in this chapter.
4.6 For a 50 kHz VCCS with $Z_S = j50$ kΩ, calculate the current nonlinearity as R_L varies from 0 to 1000 Ω.

5

Voltage Measurement and Signal Demodulation

Daniel J Nowicki

After the electrical impedance tomograph has injected the current, it must measure the voltage response from the subject. This measured voltage may range from one millivolt to over ten volts, depending on the data collection technique. In this chapter we discuss the means to overcome obstacles in signal measurement. The instrumentation necessary for this measurement includes buffers, multiplexers, amplifiers, demodulators and filters.

5.1 INTRODUCTION

There are several obstacles to overcome in measuring the voltage response. The greatest problem, and the first encountered, is the unknown source impedance across the patient's skin and skin-to-electrode interface. The common-mode voltage may be larger than the desired differential voltage. Also the frequency of the signal is too high to be directly measured with an inexpensive analog to digital converter. Finally, data collection time must be minimized.

5.2 INPUT IMPEDANCE

In Chapter 4 we showed that the advantage of a current-input/voltage-output EIT system lies in the fact that when voltage is measured at electrodes that do not carry current, the electrode contact impedance does not cause significant error. We must know this contact impedance and also the voltmeter input impedance in order to calculate the error caused by contact impedance.

Figure 2.12 shows that at 50 kHz, the skin impedance for a 1 cm^2 electrode may range from 150 to 850 Ω. Although no data for electrode contact impedance at 50 kHz are available, figure 3.1 shows that this impedance will probably be smaller than the skin impedance.

The op amps chosen as buffers should have a minimal input impedance Z_I, so that the error is less than the system's error tolerance δ (defined in Section 4.4). We can find the error resulting from the voltage divider formed by the contact impedance R_C and Z_I from

$$\delta \leq \frac{R_C}{Z_I + R_C}. \tag{5.1}$$

For a purely resistive op-amp input impedance that is much greater than R_C,

$$Z_I \geq \frac{R_C}{\delta}. \tag{5.2}$$

For example, if the system is to have 12 bit accuracy, $\delta = 1/4096$, and the contact impedance is 850 Ω, the op amp must have an input impedance greater than 3.5 MΩ.

A good op amp will have a resistive input impedance much higher than this, but at these frequencies, we must account for capacitive input impedance. Both op-amp characteristics as well as board layout contribute to this capacitance. Substituting for an input capacitance of 20 pF, $Z_I = -j160$ kΩ at 50 kHz, for $R_C = 850$ Ω, the error from equation (5.1) becomes 0.0053 at 89.7°. Separating this into real and imaginary components, $3 \cdot 10^{-5} + j0.0053$, we can see any in-phase measurements will have negligible error. Imaginary measurements will have a large error even for moderate input capacitances.

5.3 DRIVEN SHIELDS

In addition to the input capacitance from the op amp, shielded cables will have an associated capacitance. These capacitive leakage currents, as shown in figure 5.1, are another source of unwanted current through the electrode contact impedance. Along with the contact impedance, this stray capacitance will form a voltage divider with a gain of $1/(1 + j\omega R_C C)$. A 1 m coaxial cable will have a stray capacitance of about 100 pF, giving a phase shift of up to 1.5° and a gain of $0.9993 - j0.027$ when the contact impedance is 850 Ω.

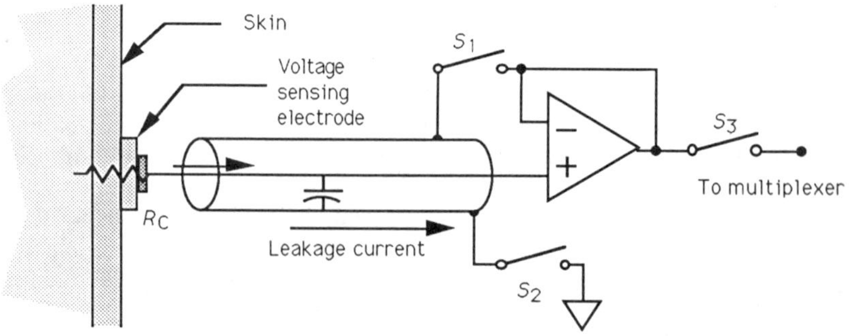

Figure 5.1 The lead from a voltage-measuring electrode. When S_1 is open and S_2 is closed, capacitive leakage current will flow to ground. When S_1 is closed and S_2 is open the shield is driven at the same potential as the center conductor so no leakage current will flow.

This gain would cause errors greater than δ if left uncorrected. By using driven shields, not unlike those discussed in Chapter 4, the effect of stray lead capacitances may be minimized. Figure 5.1 shows a means of accomplishing this with a buffer amplifier when the switch, S_1, is closed and S_2 is opened. Such a system can reduce the effective stray capacitance to about 1 pF if the op-amp open-loop gain is sufficiently high.

5.4 BUFFERS

To attain the high input impedances discussed in Section 5.2, some form of buffering is usually required early in the voltage measurement electronics. To minimize noise pickup and stray capacitance effects, we would like to physically locate the buffers as close to the patient as is practical. The extreme of this would be physical placement on the electrodes. Not only would this prove cumbersome for the patient, but the long power supply leads could pick up interference or induce oscillations if great care is not practiced in their design.

The unity gain follower shown in figure 5.2(*a*) will have a transfer function with errors associated with the finite differential-mode gain G_{DM}, and finite common-mode gain G_{CM}. More often the common-mode gain is listed instead as the common-mode rejection ratio (CMRR), where CMRR = G_{DM}/G_{CM}. Equation (5.3) shows that in an approximation for the transfer function, the error terms can be separated:

$$\frac{v_o}{v_i} = \frac{G_{DM} + \frac{1}{2}G_{CM}}{1 + G_{DM} - \frac{1}{2}G_{CM}} \approx \left(1 - \frac{1}{G_{DM}}\right)\left(1 + \frac{1}{\text{CMRR}}\right) \tag{5.3}$$

We will consider each term independently. At frequencies typical for electrical impedance tomography, 10 to 100 kHz, most op amps have an open-loop phase shift of about –90°. For instance a common, moderate bandwidth op amp, the TL074, has a specified open-loop gain of about 63 at –90°. Because of this phase shift, the differential gain based on the first term will be 1.000124 at an angle of –0.9°. For an in-phase measurement, this error will not be measurable.

Because the phase of the CMRR is closer to 0°, this error term presents a greater problem. It can easily be seen that to maintain a 12 bit accuracy the CMRR must be greater than 4096. Experimentally, at 50 kHz with an 8 pF compensation capacitance, an HA2625 had a CMRR of about 20 000.

Although a normal unity-gain follower op-amp configuration would provide adequate input impedance, as we will discuss in Section 5.7, it is also desirable to block DC currents. To accomplish this, a capacitor is sometimes placed between patient and buffer. If this were the only change, no DC bias current could flow into the positive input of the op amp, and the op amp would drift toward saturation. A resistance from positive input to ground would lower the input impedance to the value of that resistance.

A circuit to provide both DC blocking as well as high input impedance is shown in figure 5.2(*b*). At low frequencies, capacitors C_1 and C_2 act as open circuits, and no signal is passed by the buffer. As the frequency increases, C_2 acts as a short circuit so that the voltage between the resistors is the same as that at the output of the op amp. Under this condition, the voltage across R_1 is approximately zero (the voltage at the output of the op amp is nearly equal to the voltage at the positive input). With no voltage across R_1, no current will flow through it and the input impedance of the bootstrap buffer will approach infinity. At even higher frequencies, the characteristics of the op amp begin to degrade, and the input impedance begins to fall off. Figure 5.2(*c*) shows the input impedance versus frequency for the bootstrap buffer shown in figure 5.2(*b*) (Rosell *et al* 1988b).

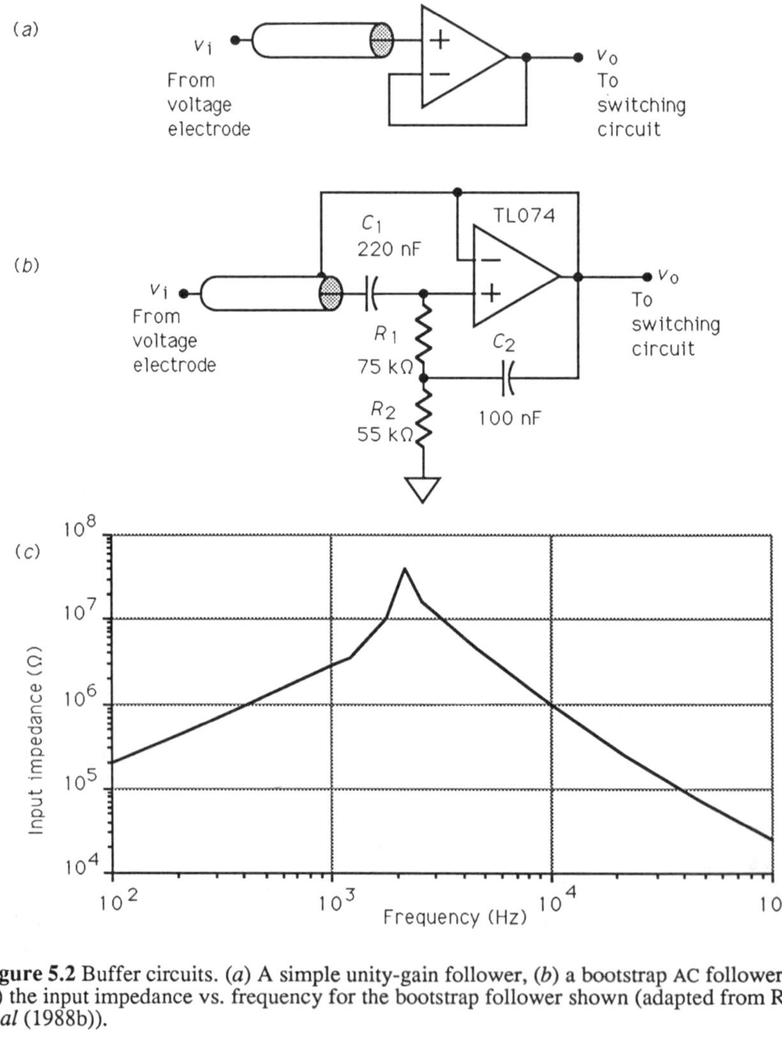

Figure 5.2 Buffer circuits. (*a*) A simple unity-gain follower, (*b*) a bootstrap AC follower, and (*c*) the input impedance vs. frequency for the bootstrap follower shown (adapted from Rosell *et al* (1988b)).

5.5 ANALOG MULTIPLEXERS (SWITCHES)

Electrical impedance tomographs are sometimes divided into types depending on the way they handle multiple-channel data. A serial device uses a single current source and a single voltage measurement circuit. Intermediate parallel devices may either use one current source and multiple measurement circuits, or multiple current sources and one measurement circuit. Finally, a fully parallel device uses multiple current sources and measurement circuits, all operating simultaneously (Rosell *et al* 1988b).

Most of the data collection methods discussed in Chapter 8 require the ability to measure the voltage between a variety of different electrodes on the subject. In order to produce a system flexible enough to do this without using one amplifier for each possible combination, one or more amplifiers are fed by an analog switching matrix. With this switching matrix, for each of the amplifier inputs we may select from any voltage-sensing electrode, a calibration source or ground.

If the switches in the switching matrix were ideal, they would have a zero on impedance and an infinite off impedance, and they would cause no errors. Because they do have finite impedances, the amplifiers could cause errors similar to those considered in equation (5.1). If no buffers are used, R_C becomes the maximal on impedance possible through the switching matrix plus the contact impedance, rather than just the contact impedance.

5.6 COMMON-MODE REJECTION

Some data collection techniques, such as the multireference method discussed in Chapter 8, may have common-mode signals in the range of volts. Because the differential signals may be as small as a few millivolts in magnitude, common-mode rejection ratios of $1000/\delta$, or about 132 dB, may be needed. If this is not achieved in the instrumentation amplifier, the common-mode signal may add an error to the differential signal we are attempting to measure.

In addition to the instrumentation amplifier, other stages of our system may convert this common-mode signal to a differential-mode signal. This is especially true for the buffer stage. For example if two buffers differ in gain by 0.01%, a 5 V common-mode signal will be converted to an undesired 0.5 mV differential signal at the buffer outputs. If the desired differential signal is 10 mV, the resulting measurement would have a 5% error.

5.7 INSTRUMENTATION AMPLIFIER

Because the actual voltages measured on the subject are so low, we must amplify them with an instrumentation amplifier such as the one shown in figure 5.3.

The first stage of the amplifier is fed by the switching matrix. To avoid error due to the switch on impedance, the amplifier must satisfy equation (4.5), where

R_C is now also due to the switches as well as the contact impedance without buffers, or just the switch impedance if buffers are used. For a typical switch on impedance of 150 Ω and contact impedance of 850 Ω, the input impedance must now be at least 4.1 MΩ. This is most easily accomplished using the buffer configuration shown in the first stage of figure 5.3.

Along with serving as a buffer, the first stage also provides some gain and common-mode rejection. While the differential gain is $1 + 2R_2/R_1$, the common-mode gain is only one. This yields a common-mode rejection ratio equal to the differential gain.

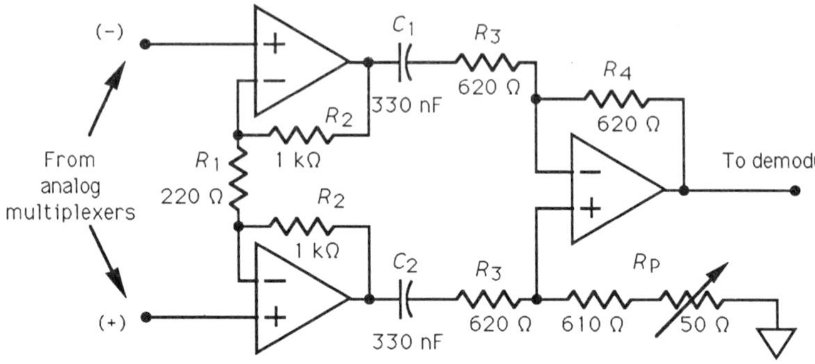

Figure 5.3 An instrumentation amplifier for amplifying a 50 kHz signal.

The second stage is a differential amplifier which also provides low-pass filtering. To get high common-mode rejection R_3/R_P should equal R_3/R_4 as nearly as possible. If this condition is met, the high-frequency differential gain of this stage is R_4/R_3.

The capacitors C_1 and C_2, along with the two resistors R_3, provide the high-pass filtering. Because capacitor values are typically difficult to match in practice, it may be difficult to match the two filters. Any difference in filter response at the operating frequency would convert the common-mode signal to a differential-mode signal which would be passed through the rest of the amplifier. For this reason, the corner frequency of the filters must be chosen sufficiently low so that the filters will have little effect at the operating frequency.

Overall the amplifier shown will have a high-pass corner frequency at 780 Hz, and a high-frequency gain of 9.9. As stated previously, this gain may be too large for some applications.

5.8 DYNAMIC RANGE

With a system that uses one electrode pair for current injection and the rest for voltage measurement, Brown and Seagar (1987) have estimated the potentials measured from various pairs on a homogeneous object. The maximal measured potential was estimated to be about $4\rho I/15D$, and the minimal potential to be about $\rho I/150D$ for an average resistivity ρ, object diameter D and injection current *I*. This yields a 40:1 dynamic range for their system. A system using multiple, adaptive currents may have an even larger dynamic range.

To maintain system accuracy over the entire dynamic range, either the DAC must have higher resolution, or the lower potentials must be normalized to the same range as the maximal potentials. For just a 40:1 range, the DAC resolution must be improved by over 5 bits. But, adding resolution dramatically increases cost and conversion time. The alternative method, normalization, may be carried out in a number of ways. A variable attenuator followed by gain would normalize the signals. Brown and Seagar (1987) use a multiplying DAC operating as a divider to get the quotient of measured to expected signals. Either of these two methods require either a good guess of the measured value, or two consecutive measurements of each potential.

5.9 DEMODULATION TECHNIQUES

The electrical impedance tomograph we are describing obtains data by measuring the effect on a carrier signal by a system. In this situation, the system is the impedance of a human body. Because we are not interested in the carrier itself, but only its amplitude, we demodulate the carrier to get the amplitude information. In this section we will discuss some hardware demodulation methods.

5.9.1 RMS-to-DC converters

Some integrated-circuit chips can be used to directly convert an AC signal to a DC signal that is a measure of its amplitude. Typically this measure is the square root of the signal mean, squared (RMS). For direct RMS-to-DC conversion in theory, the signal is squared, averaged, and then the square root is found. Because the squaring process severely limits dynamic response (Counts 1976), the actual output voltage is found by the approximation

$$v_o = \mathrm{Avg}\left(\frac{v_i^2}{v_o}\right) \approx [\mathrm{Avg}(v_i^2)]^{1/2} \qquad (5.4)$$

where v_o is the output, and v_i is the input of the converter.

Demodulators of this type are not phase sensitive even though they use multiplication. This is because the input is multiplied by itself, instead of the original oscillator output. Although these chips may have a wide bandwidth, the AD536 used by Skidmore *et al* (1987) has an accuracy of only 0.2% of the reading. This poor accuracy by itself will not present a problem as long as it is constant and linear over the entire operating range.

5.9.2 Rectifiers

Rectifiers are conceptually the simplest demodulators. They are commonly implemented by using diodes to either block the negative portion of the signal—a half-wave rectifier—or invert the negative portion of the signal—a full-wave rectifier. Once the signal has been rectified as shown in figure 5.4, converting it to DC can be accomplished simply by sending the rectified signal through a low-pass filter. After filtering, the output of a full-wave rectifier is

$$v_f = |v_m| \frac{2}{\pi} \tag{5.5}$$

where v_f is the filter output and v_m is the measured voltage. Unfortunately, along with the main carrier frequency, noise present at any other frequencies will also be rectified, and thus it will be passed through this demodulator. Henderson and Webster (1978) used a half-wave rectifier.

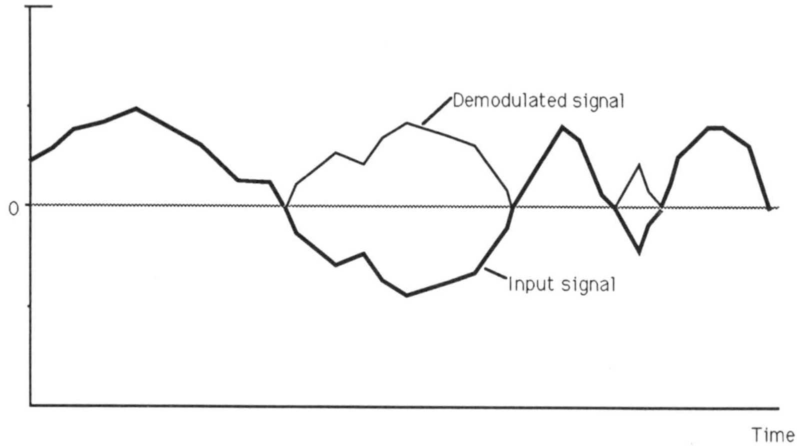

Figure 5.4 A full-wave rectified signal wave. The noise is demodulated just as is the signal we are attempting to measure.

5.9.3 Switching demodulators

A phase-sensitive demodulator uses the oscillator output to synchronously rectify the voltage signal, rather than the positive and negative swing of the measured signal itself (Webster 1978a). Demodulators of this type are also known as phase-sensitive detectors or synchronous detectors, and may be used in devices such as linear variable differential transformers.

One example of the phase-sensitive detector is the switching demodulator. Figure 5.5 shows that when the oscillator output is negative, the voltage signal is inverted. When the oscillator output is positive, the voltage signal is not inverted. In this way, the frequency components in phase with the oscillator are full-wave rectified. Frequency components in quadrature with the oscillator and at other frequencies are rejected. This is shown by the output of the demodulator after filtering

$$v_f = |v_m| \frac{2}{\pi} \cos(\phi) \tag{5.6}$$

in the case where ϕ, the phase shift between the switching function and v_m, is 90°, and thus $v_f = 0$. The rejection of noise at frequencies other than the carrier frequency is the primary advantage of any phase-sensitive demodulator.

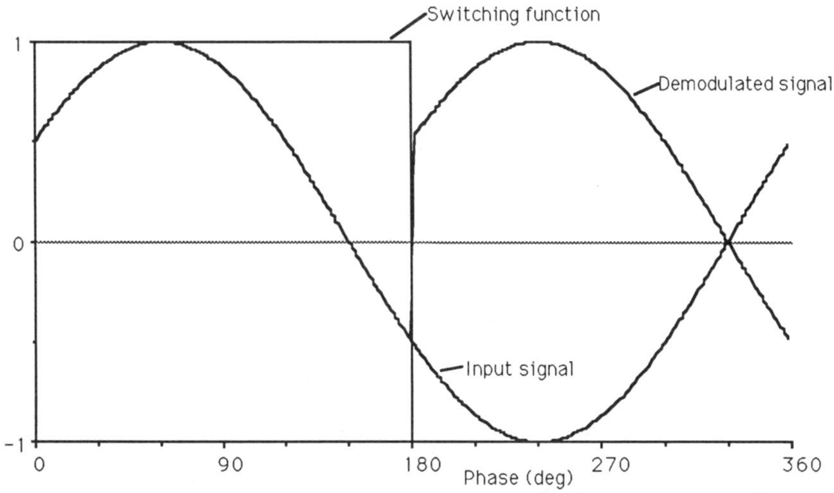

Figure 5.5 The output of a switching phase-sensitive demodulator when the input leads the switching function by 30°.

If this system has some load-dependent phase shift, one minus the cosine term will represent an error term. Therefore, for 12 bit accuracy, ϕ must change by less than 1.3° over the entire dynamic range for measurements of the real part of the impedance.

The imaginary component of the impedance may be measured in a similar manner. By shifting the oscillator output by 90° before feeding it to another demodulator, only the frequency component in quadrature will be passed after filtering. Because the cosine term is nearly one for imaginary impedance measurements, ϕ can only change by less than 0.015° if the EIT system is measuring these as well. This requirement may be impossible to achieve in actual practice.

Brown and Seagar (1987) found that the magnitude of the imaginary component was only 10% of the magnitude of the real components. Because the imaginary portion of the signal carries little information, they used a phase-sensitive demodulator to measure only the purely resistive component of the impedances.

This demodulator type may be packaged in IC form such as the AD630 (Analog Devices 1989), or built up from discrete components. The Barcelona group uses a multiplexed unity buffer/unity inverter pair, switched by using the same clock which drives their digital oscillator (Pallas-Areny 1989).

5.9.4 Multipliers

Another phase-sensitive demodulator type is the four-quadrant multiplier. Goovaerts *et al* (1988) used this demodulator. Instead of using the oscillator output as a switching function, it multiplies the signal. Figure 5.6 shows the product of the multiplication,

$$V_O V_M = |V_O||V_M| \frac{1}{2} [\cos(4\pi f_0 t + \phi) + \cos\phi]$$

and after filtering,

$$V_F = |V_O||V_M| \frac{1}{2} \cos\phi \qquad (5.7)$$

where V_O is the oscillator voltage and f_0 is the oscillator frequency. This demodulator has the same dependence on phase shift as the phase-sensitive demodulator but, as we will show in the next section, it has the disadvantage of being more susceptible to fluctuations in the amplitude of V_O.

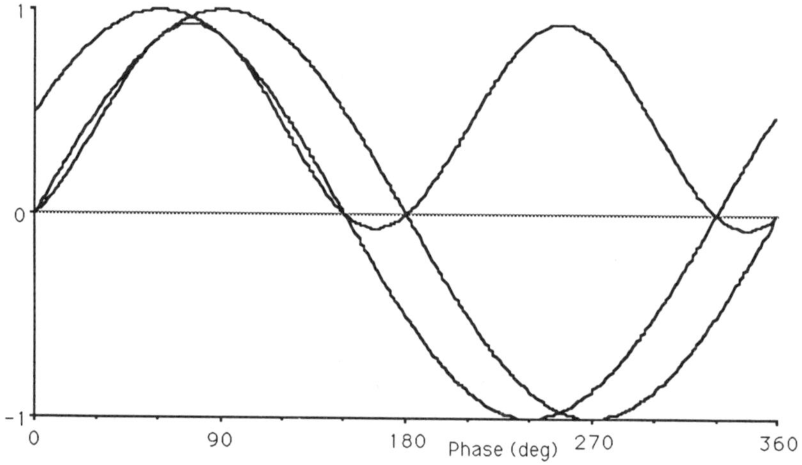

Figure 5.6 Output of a multiplying demodulator when one input leads the other by 30°.

5.9.5 Noise considerations

Nonrandom noise for different demodulation techniques can sometimes be predicted mathematically given certain conditions. The error contribution from amplitude jitter and harmonic distortion in the oscillator will be considered in this section.

As the name implies, a multiplying demodulator simply multiplies two signals. In our application these signals are the oscillator reference, and an amplified version of the voltage response measured from the body. If the oscillator amplitude varies by ε from the desired value A, we find the system's output by multiplying the new reference, $A(1 + \varepsilon)$, by the amplifier's output. If the measured response under ideal conditions is changed by a linear multiplier G, the amplifier output will be $AG(1 + \varepsilon)$, giving an output of

$$|V_O V_M| = A(1+\varepsilon)\cdot AG(1+\varepsilon) = A^2G(1+2\varepsilon+\varepsilon^2) \approx A^2G(1+2\varepsilon) \qquad (5.8)$$

because $\varepsilon \ll 1$. From this result, we can see the output is incorrect by 2ε from the desired result of A^2G.

The action of a switching demodulator can be thought of as a multiplication of the amplified voltage response and a squared, normalized reference. Thus the output under the same conditions would be

$$|V_S V_M| = AG(1+\varepsilon) \qquad (5.9)$$

or a difference of ε from the desired value of AG.

The second issue we must consider is the harmonic distortion that can be attributed to the oscillator. Murphy and Rolfe (1988) describe the effects of oscillator distortion on system accuracy for a switching demodulator. For an oscillator with a distorted output V_O, we may write

$$V_O = \cos(\omega_0 t) + \sum_{n=2}^{\infty} C_n \cos(n\omega_0 t) \qquad (5.10)$$

where ω_0 is the desired oscillator frequency, n is the harmonic number and C_n is the amplitude coefficient of that harmonic. The voltage measured from the patient may then be

$$V_M = \alpha\cos(\omega_0 t + \theta_1) + \sum_{n=2}^{\infty} \beta_n C_n \cos(n\omega_0 t + \theta_n)$$

where α and β_n are the attenuation factors for the fundamental and other harmonics respectively, and θ_1 and θ_n are the phase shifts for each of the harmonics.

For a multiplying demodulator, the two signals V_O and V_M are multiplied together. No frequency terms but DC are present after the low-pass filtering necessary in this type of demodulator. This leaves an output of

$$\overline{V_O V_M} = \frac{\alpha}{2}\cos\theta_1 + \sum_{n=2}^{\infty} \frac{\beta_n}{2} C_n^2 \cos\theta_n \Rightarrow \frac{1}{2}\left(1 + \sum_{n=2}^{\infty} C_n^2\right)$$

for the worst case when $\theta_n = 0$ and $\alpha = \beta_n = 1$. This gives an error of

$$\sum_{n=2}^{\infty} C_n^2. \qquad (5.11)$$

A good switching demodulator will have a switching function resembling a perfect square wave, as long as the oscillator output passes cleanly through the threshold region. Using Fourier series, we can find this switching function V_S, as

$$V_S = A\frac{4}{\pi}\sum_{n=1}^{\infty}\frac{1}{n}\sin(n\frac{\pi}{2})\cos(n\omega_0 t)$$

$$= A\frac{4}{\pi}\left[\cos(\omega_0 t) - \frac{1}{3}\cos(3\omega_0 t) + \frac{1}{5}\cos(5\omega_0 t) - \frac{1}{7}\cos(7\omega_0 t) + \ldots\right] \quad (5.12)$$

After multiplying this by the same distorted signal as above, V_M, we find the demodulator output signal after filtering as

$$\overline{V_S V_M} = \frac{A4\alpha}{\pi}\cos\theta_1 + \frac{A4}{\pi}\sum_{n=3}^{\infty}\frac{\beta_n C_n}{n}\cos\theta_n \Rightarrow \frac{A4}{\pi}\left[1 + \sum_{n=3}^{\infty}\frac{C_n}{n}\right] \quad n \text{ odd}$$

again, for the worst case when $\theta_n = 0$ and $\alpha = \beta_n = 1$. This gives an error of

$$\sum_{n=3}^{\infty}\frac{C_n}{n} \quad n \text{ odd.} \quad (5.13)$$

A third noise consideration is demodulator rejection of random noise from any other sources. Because these noise sources are almost never synchronized with the master oscillator, the demodulated result that they produce will not be a DC value. Instead, their result will be the image frequencies produced when multiplying two sinusoidal signals. An oscillator frequency f_0, and a noise frequency f_N, will produce two new signal at $|f_0 + f_N|$ and $|f_0 - f_N|$. As long as these new signals fall outside of the pass band of the low-pass filter after the demodulator, they will not cause a problem, but for noise signals near the oscillator frequency, one of the image frequencies may be passed through a normal filter with little attenuation. For example, the resulting frequencies from a 35 kHz noise source and an electrical impedance tomograph operating at 50 kHz using a multiplying demodulator will be 15 and 85 kHz. A low-pass filter with a corner frequency at about 15 kHz will block most of the 85 kHz result, but only attenuate the lower frequency result by a factor of two. For this reason, care must be taken when using a phase-sensitive demodulator near a noise source such as some computer display screens.

A switching demodulator will have the same noise problem as a pure multiplying demodulator along with additional sensitivity to noise at $3f_0$, $5f_0$, $7f_0$ etc. This is due to the presence of these frequencies in the multiplication.

5.9.6 Digital demodulation

Smith *et al* (1989) described a system for collecting and processing resistivity images at 25 frames per second. A significant source of noise was shown to be the phase-sensitive detector. It was shown that a matched filter design provides the maximal SNR. Though this can be implemented by either analog or digital techniques, they found that the digital demodulator using a TMS 32020 DSP gave a SNR much closer to the theoretical value than the analog design.

Their system uses parallel data collection using 16 electrodes to improve the SNR. By using a parallel instead of a serial system, they expected an improvement of $13^{1/2}$ in SNR since the integration time constant can be increased by 13 (ie 16 – 3). From measurements on a cylindrical tank, they showed a 20 dB improvement in SNR of the digital parallel data collection system when compared with the serial analog design.

5.10 FILTERS

After demodulation by one of the above full-wave methods, the signal will have a fundamental ripple frequency at twice the operating frequency. In order to sample the voltage, this frequency must be filtered out. Even RMS-to-DC converters will have some ripple in their output which may be larger than δ, and thus will require filtering.

A first-order filter will have a frequency response which decreases with a slope of –1, as shown in figure 5.7. Thus, to attain an attenuation of δ, the corner frequency of the filter must be δ times the frequency out of the demodulator. For a 50 kHz oscillator, the ripple frequency will be 100 kHz, and the filter corner frequency f_c, must be 24.4 Hz to maintain 12 bit accuracy. Higher order filters will have a slope of $-n$, where n is the order of the filter. The corner frequency for these higher order filters will be

$$f_c = 2f_0(\delta)^{1/n}. \tag{5.14}$$

Under the same conditions, a fourth-order filter would require f_c = 12.5 kHz.

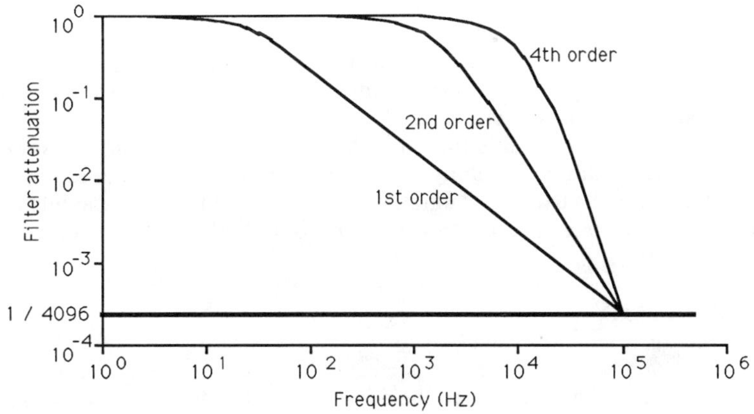

Figure 5.7 The gain of Butterworth low-pass filters with 1, 2 and 4 poles. Each has a corner frequency that will attenuate a 100 kHz ripple frequency by a factor of $1/2^{12}$.

Filter settling time is easily the primary limitation on measurement speed. The step response for an nth order Butterworth filter is

$$\frac{v_o}{v_i} = 1 - e^{-\omega_c t}\left(1 + \omega_c t + \frac{\omega_c{}^2 t^2}{2!} + \ldots + \frac{(\omega_c t)^{(n-1)}}{(n-1)!}\right) \qquad (5.15)$$

For a first-order system, this reduces to a simple exponential equation:

$$\frac{v_o}{v_i} = 1 - e^{-\omega_c t}. \qquad (5.16)$$

For the above conditions, it would take 54.3 ms before the filter output settles to within 1/4096 of the true voltage. A second-order filter on the other hand would only require 1.1 ms and a fourth-order filter 190 μs. To measure 32 voltages, a system using one of the above filters would take 1.74 s, 35.2 ms or 6.08 ms respectively. If the time to take the measurements is a significant part of one heartbeat, images of the thorax will become blurred.

Although this discussion has been limited to Butterworth filters, other filters will have comparable attenuations and time lags, but they may be optimized for certain characteristics. For instance, although a Bessel filter will have less attenuation for a given corner frequency than a Butterworth or Chebyshev filter, the Bessel filter will settle to the correct value more quickly than either of these other filters. This is because a Bessel filter has very little ringing after a step input.

Adaptive methods will require even longer times to acquire a complete data set. One method of taking data faster would be the use of more than one demodulator. Such a system was used by Pallas-Areny (1989).

5.11 INTEGRATORS

As discussed in the section on filters, a filter with adequate stop-band rejection will also have a long step response. In most systems this becomes the dominant factor in slowing data collection speed.

By using an integrator this time may be cut to as short as one period of the driving function, although usually ten or more periods are used to reduce noise. Pallas-Areny (1989) uses an integrator following a switching demodulator, and Eyuboglu (1989) uses an integrator following a multiplying demodulator.

5.12 SUMMARY

In this chapter we have presented the components that comprise the second half of an electrical impedance tomograph, namely, the voltage-measuring section. To achieve high input impedance, buffers are used as early as possible in the circuit. The buffered channels may then be multiplexed so that only one amplifier, demodulator, etc. is needed. A simple instrumentation amplifier provides initial gain and may feed some form of normalization circuit. Finally, various demodulator schemes and some of their advantages were then discussed, along with some filter considerations.

5.13 STUDY QUESTIONS

5.1 Estimate the stray capacitance of 1 m of shielded cable and calculate its impedance at 50 kHz.

5.2 Estimate the common-mode voltage, and then using the result of the previous problem, estimate the common-mode-to-differential conversion factor when one voltmeter lead has a contact impedance of 100 Ω and the other 200 Ω.

5.3 Give the relation for minimal Z_I if R_C is imaginary instead of real.

5.4 List the specification for CMRR for the voltmeter.

5.5 Estimate the the differential signal resulting from a common-mode voltage on the patient if the contact impedance were 1 kΩ and the shield capacitances differed by 5% from a nominal value of 150 pF.

5.6 Describe the operation of a multiplier demodulator and list its advantages and disadvantages.

5.7 Describe the operation of a phase-sensitive demodulator and lists its advantages and disadvantages.

5.8 Calculate the corner frequency of a second-order low-pass filter that will reduce the ripple of a 50 kHz demodulated signal to 12 bit accuracy.

5.9 For the filter of the previous problem, calculate the time to measure 32 serial voltages.

6

Electrical Safety

Ali Ghahary

Any medical electrical equipment must pass very strict safety requirements, and the electrical impedance tomography (EIT) system is no exception. The specifications set for medical electrical equipment range from requirements to ensure proper and accurate operation of the machine to ones that ensure the safety of the patient. This chapter will describe how to meet one of the safety requirements for the EIT system: the limit imposed on the currents that flow through the patient via any leads connected to him. For the EIT system the patient-connected leads are the 32 current source leads and the 32 voltage-sensing leads.

6.1 INTRODUCTION

In defining the safety requirements of the system, we will follow the guidelines set by four organizations. These are: National Fire Protection Association (NFPA), Association for the Advancement of Medical Instrumentation (AAMI), Underwriters Laboratories (UL), and International Electrotechnical Commission (IEC). The first three organizations are responsible for setting the USA standards for patient lead current limits. The IEC, on the other hand, is responsible for setting the standards for many countries throughout the world, not including the USA and Canada (Lipschultz 1989). All four organizations have similar standards regarding currents flowing through patient leads, although each one uses different terminology.

6.2 CLASSIFICATION OF CURRENTS IN PATIENT LEADS

The currents flowing through the patient leads in the EIT system are of two types. The first type is the currents needed for normal use of the system, which consist mainly of the 50 kHz currents generated by the 32 current-source electrodes, and amplifier bias currents. The second type is any lead leakage currents, which should ideally be zero. Lead leakage currents are divided into three categories by National Fire Protection Association (1987). These are: leakage current from patient leads to ground, AC isolation (risk) current, and leakage current between patient leads. Figure 6.1 (*a–c*) shows the situations where these three currents exist.

Figure 6.1(*a*) shows that if a patient comes in contact with ground, a lead to ground leakage current can flow through the patient lead and his body to ground if there is any leakage impedance Z_L between the patient-connected circuitry and the hot conductor of the power system. A large Z_L is desirable to minimize the leakage current.

Figure 6.1(*b*) shows that if a patient touches 120 V, a leakage current, called AC isolation or risk current, can flow from the 120 V line, through the patient and Z_L, to ground. Z_L, in this case, is the leakage impedance between the circuitry connected to the patient's body and ground. As in the case of lead-to-ground leakage current, a large Z_L is desirable to minimize the risk current.

Finally, figure 6.1(*c*) shows that it is possible for an instrument to have a current flow between two of its leads through the patient. This current can either be a low-frequency leakage current or a current required for the normal operation of the system. In case of the EIT system, the normal use current is either the amplifier bias current or a 50 kHz current injected through the patient between any two patient leads. This 50 kHz current may be as high as 5 mA_{RMS}.

Figure 6.2 compares the terminologies and maximal safe limits set by the four organizations mentioned earlier for the currents described above (Association for the Advancement of Medical Instrumentation 1985, International Electrotechnical Commission 1977, National Fire Protection Association 1987, Underwriters Laboratories 1976).

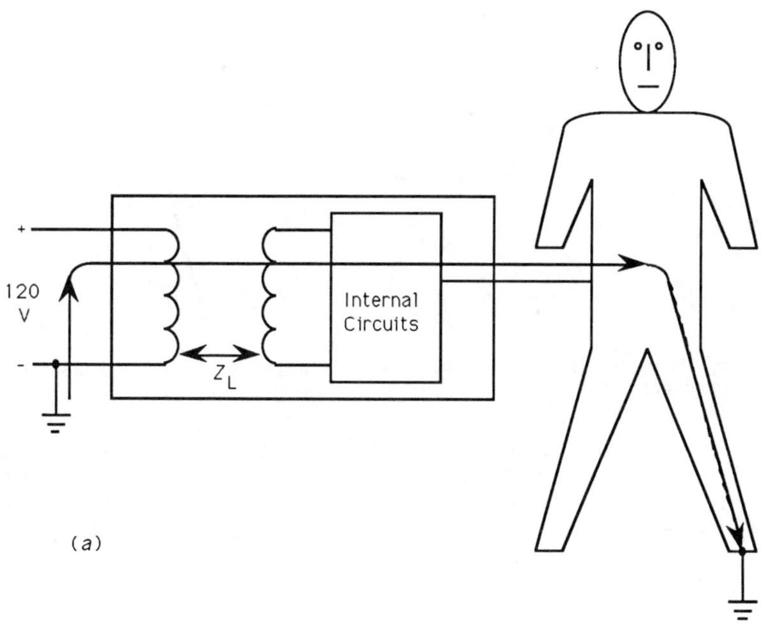

(*a*)

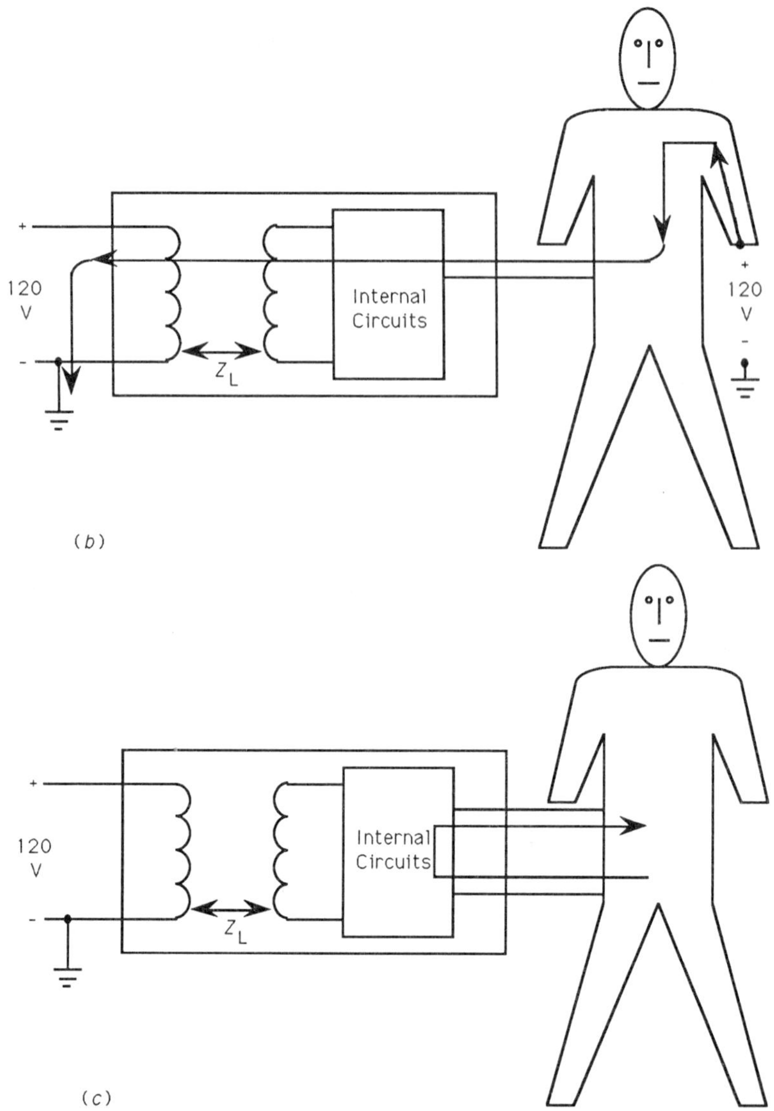

Figure 6.1 Patient lead currents, (*a*) lead-to-gound leakage, (*b*) AC isolation, and (*c*) current between patient leads.

In order to meet the standards set forth by the four organizations, all medical electrical equipment must have lead currents lower than the limits indicated in figure 6.2. The instruments must be tested under all possible combinations of the following operating conditions: with the instrument on and off, with the ground wire broken and intact, and with the applied power polarity forward and reversed. The interested reader can find more detailed information in the individual organizations' standards.

Type of current	NFPA	AAMI	UL[a]	IEC
Leakage, figure 6.1(*a*)	Lead-to-ground leakage 10 (100)	Patient-Patient source connection 10 (50)	10 (50)	Patient leakage 10 (100)
Leakage, figure 6.1(*b*)	AC isolation or risk 10[b] (N/A)	Patient-Patient sink connection 10[b] (N/A)	10[b] (N/A)	Patient leakage 10 (N/A)
Leakage, figure 6.1(*c*)	Leakage between leads 10 (50)	Patient-Patient source connection 10 (50)	10 (50)	Patient auxiliary 10 (100)
Injected figure 6.1(*c*)	Leakage between leads 10 (50)	Patient-Patient source connection 10 (50)	10 (50)	Patient auxiliary 10 (100)

[a] Multiply all the UL values by 1.4 for DC quantities.

[b] This value is the maximal limit at the input terminals of the device. When there is a connection cable between the instrument and the patient, the current at the patient end of the connection may be up to 20 μA to allow for some leakage to the cable shield.

Figure 6.2 Comparison of patient current terminologies and limits in microamperes.

Figure 6.2 shows that the four organizations differ slightly in the way they classify the currents; however, they all impose similar maximal limits under comparable conditions. The limits stated in figure 6.2 are for signals at frequencies less than 1 kHz. For signals greater than 1 kHz, the limit is multiplied by the frequency, in kilohertz, up to a multiplier of 100. The numbers outside the parentheses apply to equipment with patient leads isolated from the power lines. These are instruments used on a patient with a direct connection to his heart. The numbers inside the parentheses are for instruments with nonisolated patient leads; therefore, they are less conservative limits.

The increased value of the IEC Patient auxiliary current (100 μA) is intended to permit the design of simple equipment for impedance plethysmography and applies only to currents having a frequency of not less than 0.1 Hz. Thus at 50 kHz, we can pass (100 μA)(50) = 5 mA of normal current injected by the current source electrodes.

We will use the NFPA terminology to refer to all three types of leakage current whenever possible. The rest of this chapter will focus on how the proposed EIT system developed by the Wisconsin group will attempt to meet the above safety requirements. Generally, each type of leakage current can be limited by inserting an isolation barrier in the current path. The normal use current, on the other hand, is already at a safe value as long as the instrument does not malfunction. For the amplifier bias currents, the safety limit is 10 μA, which is much larger than their actual value.

6.3 FUNCTIONAL BLOCK DIAGRAM

Figure 6.3 shows a block diagram of the whole EIT system. A microcomputer controls the whole system through a Digital I/O board. It sends commands via 24 digital lines to a digital control board. The digital control board can select any combination of 32 current source electrodes through each of which it can send up to 5 mA of current into the body at 50 kHz. It can also select any two out of 32 voltage-sensing electrodes in order to make a differential 50 kHz voltage measurement from the body. The differential voltage then goes through an instrumentation amplifier, and a phase-sensitive demodulator, where it is converted into a direct-current (DC) voltage and fed into the microcomputer for further processing. There is also an oscillator which generates a reference 50 kHz signal to be used by the current sources and the phase-sensitive demodulator.

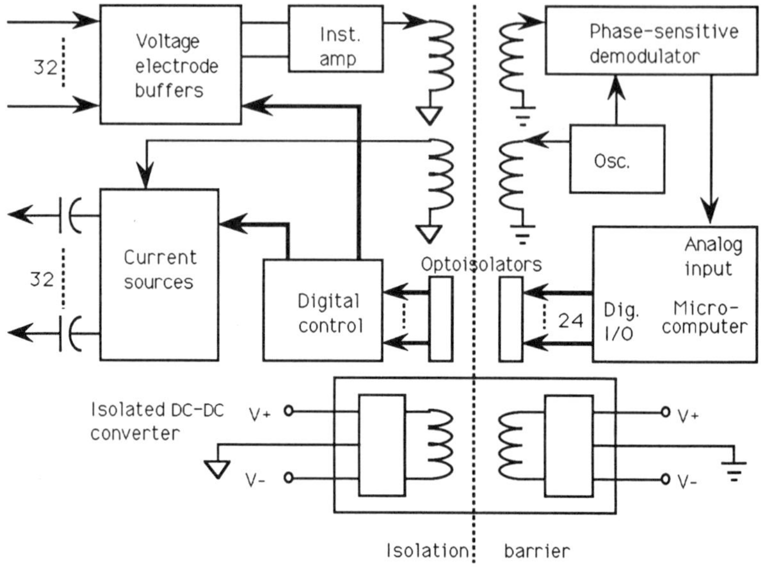

Figure 6.3 The proposed Wisconsin EIT system uses optoisolators to transmit digital signals and transformers for analog signals and power. Bold lines indicate digital control.

The dashed line from the top to the bottom of figure 6.3 shows where an isolation barrier will be placed in the present EIT system. This barrier controls the lead-to-ground leakage and the AC isolation (risk) currents. For controlling the leakage current between patient leads, decoupling capacitors are used, the circuit is also protected from power line interference.

The nonisolated circuitry in the system is powered by a DC power supply which is driven by the line voltage. This DC supply also drives an isolated DC-to-DC converter which powers all the isolated circuitry.

6.4 LEAD-TO-GROUND LEAKAGE AND RISK CURRENTS

If we want to limit lead-to-ground leakage and risk currents, the EIT system should not connect any part of the patient's body to ground during normal operation of the instrument. However, any medical electrical equipment which makes voltage measurements from the body must have a common reference point on the body. All the circuitry that contacts the patient must therefore be referenced to a common point isolated from earth ground.

In the EIT system, the microcomputer is referenced to earth ground. Hence, at some point between the computer and the circuits attached to the body, there needs to be an isolation barrier. On one side of the barrier is the isolated circuitry which connects to the patient, and on the other side is the grounded circuitry which connects to the microcomputer. This isolation barrier needs to limit any leakage current while faithfully transmitting the digital and the 50 kHz analog data.

6.4.1 Lead-to-ground leakage current

From figure 6.1(*a*), the worst case for the lead-to-ground leakage current is when we assume the patient resistance to be negligible, which is a reasonable assumption if the patient leads directly contact the tissue below the skin. In this case, the loop for the lead-to-ground leakage consists only of the line voltage in series with the leakage impedance Z_L. Therefore, the minimal required impedance across the isolation barrier between the circuit common and earth ground, assuming an instrument with isolated leads, is:

$$Z_L = \frac{V_L}{10\ \mu\text{A}} \tag{6.1}$$

where V_L is the RMS line voltage. In the USA, where V_L is 120 V at 60 Hz, the minimal Z_L is 12 MΩ. On the other hand, in Europe, where V_L is 240 V at 50 Hz, the minimal Z_L is 24 MΩ.

This leakage impedance is mainly capacitive. Therefore, the maximal allowable leakage capacitance, C_L, from one side of the isolation barrier to the other is 221 pF in the USA and 133 pF in Europe. This maximal limit applies to the total allowable capacitance across the isolation barrier in figure 6.3, including the two isolation transformers, the optoisolators, the DC–DC converter, and any other leakage capacitance not accounted for in this discussion.

6.4.2 AC isolation current

The AC isolation current limit places the same kind of constraints on the isolation barrier between the isolated common and earth ground. Since the isolated circuitry common point is attached to the patient's body, the worst case to consider for limiting the AC isolation current is when the isolated common itself touches the line voltage; that is, when the isolated common is raised to the line voltage with respect to earth ground. In this case, the minimal series impedance Z_L needed between the isolated common and earth ground is the same as that needed to limit the lead-to-ground leakage current, which is 12 MΩ for USA and 24 MΩ for Europe.

Assuming the leakage impedance across the isolation barrier to be capacitive, the maximal allowable total leakage capacitance across this barrier can be 221 pF for the USA and 131 pF for Europe. In order to meet the safety requirements in Europe as well as the United States, we choose the lower maximal limit of 131 pF for C_L.

6.4.3 Common means of isolation

The two most common means of isolation are transformers and optical isolators/couplers. Usually, an optical isolator is cheaper than a transformer; and therefore it is the preferred choice. However, for some applications an optical isolator cannot be used. In the following paragraphs we discuss the possibilities for using both types of isolators for the EIT system.

Optical couplers provide excellent isolation across the barrier; however they have limited bandwidth for analog signals. In addition, it is probably very difficult to keep good amplitude accuracy across an optical coupler for analog data without using digital coding techniques. An optical isolator therefore probably cannot be used for the transmission of analog data in the EIT system since the present system operates at 50 kHz and it requires 0.02% transmission accuracy. The digital data, on the other hand, do not need such a high transmission accuracy, so optical isolators can be used very easily to isolate the digital lines feeding the digital control board.

For the transmission of analog data, isolation transformers should be used. However, most standard isolation transformers have a leakage capacitance of greater than 131 pF between the primary and the secondary. Hence, the manufacturer of the instrument may have to custom build the isolation transformers if he wants low-leakage transformers which also have a high coupling coefficient from the primary to the secondary.

6.4.4 Choosing the points of isolation

In choosing the points of isolation for the EIT system, we should consider the following. First, every effort should be made to put the isolation barriers at points where the system performance would be the least disturbed while breaking the smallest number of signal paths. Second, the signal paths to be broken by an isolation barrier should be low-power paths.

We chose the following points of isolation: for the digital signals, the most logical place to isolate the microcomputer from the rest of the circuitry was right at the point where the signals leave the computer. Since the A/D and Digital I/O boards are inside the computer, the best point of isolation would be right at the output of the Digital I/O board. Figure 6.3 shows that 24 optoisolators are then needed between the Digital I/O board and the Digital control board.

For the analog signals, we chose two points of isolation. The first one is between the instrumentation amplifier and the phase-sensitive demodulator, and the second point is between the oscillator and the current sources, as shown in figure 6.3. At both of these points, the analog signal is AC, and an isolation transformer could be placed directly into the circuit. Any transformer placed at these points would not have to handle more than 1/4 W of power.

Optoisolators have a finite rise and fall time, which limits the rate at which they can process digital data. In order to make sure all the digital data are transmitted correctly, any pulse from the Digital I/O board of the microcomputer must have a width which is greater than the response time of the optoisolator. Therefore, the data rate of the optoisolator is the maximal rate at which the digital I/O board may operate. Commercially, optoisolators with data rates of up to 10 Mbit/s are available (Hewlett Packard 1988).

Isolation transformers also have some nonideal behavior associated with their transfer characteristics from the primary to the secondary; however, their exact gain is not important, as long as it is stable. The gain of the transformer from the primary to secondary must remain constant to within 0.02% for the duration of one set of current injections and voltage measurements, which is less than 1 s. It is very unlikely that the gain of a transformer would change by an appreciable amount during 1 s. As long as an isolation transformer has a small enough leakage capacitance between the primary and the secondary and a reasonable magnetic coupling, it is acceptable for use in the EIT system.

6.5 CURRENT BETWEEN PATIENT LEADS

The only patient leads with the possibility of an appreciable current flowing through them are the current-source electrodes. The voltage-sensing electrodes are buffered by high-input-impedance op amps and they conduct only a small amount of bias current.

6.5.1 Types of current between leads

There are three sources of possible currents flowing in the current source electrodes. The first and most important current is the 50 kHz reconstruction current injected intentionally into the patient. This current is limited by the microcomputer to a safe value during the normal operation of the instrument. As long as the software runs properly, the total RMS current flowing through all the current-source electrodes and the patient will not exceed 5 mA, which is the maximal safe value allowed according to the standards cited above. However, the hardware of the EIT system is capable of putting out 5 mA RMS current through each current source, resulting in possible current levels of much higher than 5 mA at 50 kHz. Should there be a malfunction in the operation of the system, the hardware could inject currents into the patient which would violate the safety standards. Therefore, a means of hardware limiting the 50 kHz injected current should be provided in the system. Currently, the Wisconsin EIT system does not have such a hardware protection, and this subject needs further study.

The second type of current is any DC component caused by the saturation of the current source electrode op amps. This current should not be present under normal operating conditions. However, when the instrument is first turned on or in case of any malfunction in the software or the hardware, the current-source op amps could saturate and inject an appreciable amount of DC current through the patient. Considering just two of the current sources, if one of them saturates to +15 V and the other to –15 V, and there is roughly 1 kΩ of patient interface resistance between them, then approximately 30 mA of DC current could flow through the patient, which would be dangerous.

The third type of current can be caused by power line interference on the circuit either through leakage capacitive paths or through electromagnetic interference. If there is some power line frequency voltage induced at the input of a current source, then a corresponding current will appear at the output.

Depending on the magnitude of induced noise and the voltage to current gain of the current source, this line frequency current could become larger than the maximal limit allowed by the safety standards.

6.5.2 Possible solutions

We have considered some possible solutions for limiting the DC and the power line frequency currents between the patient leads. This section will describe the results of our study.

The first possibility is the placement of series capacitors between the current source op amps and the patient. These series capacitors could block the DC component and limit the low-frequency, line-power-induced component of the current. In order to limit the line frequency current to a value below the maximal limit allowed by the safety standards, the series capacitors must be small. However, any small capacitor in series with the patient at the output of the current source will exhibit an appreciable series impedance at the reconstruction frequency of 50 kHz and degrade the system performance. It would be impossible to have a capacitor which is small enough to limit the line-frequency-induced current to a safe value but at the same time large enough to not have a significant impedance at the 50 kHz frequency of operation.

The second solution considered is the placement of transformers in series with the current source outputs. These transformers would block any DC component of lead currents and they would also provide isolation of all the current source electrodes from each other. However, they also have some problems associated with them. First, each transformer has a finite magnetizing inductance which would lower the output impedance of and at the same time load the current source. Second, all the 32 transformers would have to be matched for gain and phase shift from the primary to the secondary so that they would not introduce errors in the reconstruction process. This requirement is extremely difficult to meet.

After considering the above points, we recommend the following measures to be taken in order to limit the DC and low-frequency patient lead currents. For limiting the DC current, put a large blocking capacitor, on the order of 100 nF, in series with each current source electrode. For limiting the power line frequency currents in the patient leads, provide good insulation of the current source boards from the line voltage and at the same time provide a good electromagnetic shield around the whole instrument.

6.6 POWER SUPPLY REQUIREMENT

As we mentioned earlier, the isolated circuitry in our EIT system will run from an isolated DC-to-DC converter which supplies ±15 V output. This converter will in turn be powered by an AC-to-DC converter which runs from line power. The AC-DC converter will also power all the nonisolated circuits in the EIT system.

We would like to estimate how much power the isolated DC-to-DC converter will have to deliver by reviewing the power requirements of the isolated circuitry. For detailed descriptions of all the hardware please refer to Chapters 4 and 5.

There are 32 current sources each of which requires 15 mA; a buffer board which needs 20 mA, and the rest of the isolated circuitry requires roughly 80 mA. These numbers are all estimates based on experimental measurements. The total current required is then approximately 600 mA. To obtain the power requirement, this current needs to be multiplied by 30 V (±15 V) resulting in a value of 18 W.

Therefore, the isolated power supply needs to supply at least 18 W; however, we will impose a safety margin and make the power requirement 36 W. Recall that the capacity of the isolated supply across the isolation barrier has to be low enough to limit the lead-to-ground and AC isolation currents.

6.7 POSSIBLE SOURCES FOR SPECIFIC PARTS

In this section, we will discuss some of the isolation components which are commercially available at the present time. For each type of component, one commercial source will be named. The vendors mentioned are not necessarily the only or even the best sources for these parts. They are just mentioned to serve as a starting point to anyone interested in building an EIT system.

6.7.1 Isolation transformers

Of the three isolation components, the isolation transformer is the simplest one to custom build. In fact, many designers may prefer to build this component rather than buying it. However, for those who prefer to buy commercial transformers, Pico Electronics, Inc. in Mt. Vernon, NY is one possible vendor.

Pico makes a variety of transformers for many applications (Pico Electronics Inc. 1988). Many of their transformers meet the maximal allowable leakage capacitance requirement from the primary to secondary; however, there is no specification regarding this capacitance value given in their catalog. If a designer needs to be guaranteed a certain maximal capacitance between the transformer windings, he can obtain such a part from Pico through special ordering.

6.7.2 Optical isolators

Several companies supply reliable, digital optoisolators at a low cost. Therefore we recommend that any designer in need of an optoisolator buy one rather than attempting to build it himself. One of the most reputable suppliers of these components with a wide selection of parts is Hewlett Packard (1988).

6.7.3 Isolated DC-to-DC converter

The isolated DC-to-DC converter is the most expensive and complicated of the three discussed. In addition, there are very few companies which make standard power supplies suitable for medical instrumentation. Therefore, most manufacturers of medical equipment build their own custom power supplies for the patient-connected circuitry.

Condor DC Power Supplies, Inc. is one of the few suppliers of isolated standard power supplies for medical equipment. They have a wide selection of DC-to-DC converters with output power of up to approximately 40 W (Condor DC Power Supplies Inc. 1988).

6.8 OTHER GROUPS' SOLUTIONS

Two other prominent groups are conducting research on the same subject. D C Barber and B H Brown are the primary researchers for the Sheffield group in Royal Hallamshire Hospital, Sheffield, England. J C Newell, D G Gisser, and D Isaacson are the primary researchers for the group at Rensselaer Polytechnic Institute, Troy, NY. This section briefly discusses how they have attempted to meet the electrical safety requirements of their systems.

6.8.1 Sheffield Group

The Sheffield group has an EIT system quite different from the one we have proposed at Wisconsin (Brown and Seagar 1987). Their system uses 16 electrodes, and it uses the same electrodes for current injection as well as voltage measurement by time multiplexing these events during a measurement cycle. The current is injected into the patient from a single current source through successive pairs of electrodes selected by a multiplexer.

Even though the Sheffield group uses a different EIT system, they employ similar measures as the ones we have proposed with regard to patient safety. For limiting the lead-to-ground leakage current and AC isolation current, they use 16 optoisolators and two transformers to isolate the patient-connected circuitry from earth ground. With regard to currents between patient leads they also use blocking capacitors as we have previously described.

The reconstruction current for the Sheffield system is 5 mA RMS at 50 kHz, which is the maximal limit imposed by the safety standards. One advantage of the Sheffield system over ours in terms of patient safety is that since they only use one current source and inject current at one point, there is a very small chance of injecting a very large 50 kHz current in case of any equipment malfunction. They do not therefore have to consider a hardware limit on the reconstruction current.

For limiting any possible DC current in the electrodes, the Sheffield group uses large DC blocking capacitors in series with all the patient leads. Finally, for minimizing any power line interference, they have mounted the patient-connected circuitry inside a grounded shield with PVC mounts. They have adequately insulated the critical circuits from capacitive as well as electromagnetic interference from the power line.

6.8.2 Rensselaer Group

The Rensselaer group uses a reconstruction concept more similar to our system (Newell *et al* 1988). They use 32 electrodes, each of which has a programmable current source. At any time, one of the electrodes can be connected to a voltmeter for a voltage measurement. The whole system is controlled by a microcomputer.

With regard to lead-to-ground leakage and AC isolation currents, the Rensselaer group has decided to isolate the whole system including the microcomputer from earth ground through a 1 kVA line isolation transformer. In their newer designs, they are planning to use optoisolators to further isolate the computer from the rest of the electronics.

The Rensselaer system injects a 15 kHz current at amplitudes of up to 5 mA. For their frequency of operation, 5 mA is more than the allowable safe limit for certain operating conditions according to the safety standards mentioned earlier. If the instrument is to have isolated patient leads, the Rensselaer system violates all of the four safety standards. If the instrument is not to have isolated patient leads, then this system violates the standards set by the IEC.

We do not have information on how they have attempted to block any DC current flowing through the electrodes or limit the low-frequency current induced by power line interference.

6.9 CONCLUSIONS

In this chapter, we have reviewed some of the safety concerns about the patient-connected electrodes. The standards described have used very conservative limits for the maximal allowable currents in the patient leads. However, the health care facilities and the medical instruments industry still follow these standards. In order to relax these conservative limits, more research needs to be conducted in this area.

We have not discussed how to protect the equipment from damage if a defibrillator is applied to the patient. If the EIT system is to be used on any patient with any possible need for defibrillation, the designer will have to provide protection circuitry for all the parts connected to the patient. For the EIT system, a protection scheme similar to one used for commercial electrocardiographs would be acceptable.

6.10 STUDY QUESTIONS

6.1 For each of the leakage currents in figure 6.1, describe in your own words the origin of the current, and how it might be blocked.

6.2 List the specifications for an instrument so that it would pass every safety test in this chapter. See figure 6.2.

6.3 Design a test for each of these requirements.

6.4 Look up the specifications on any available optoisolator, and discuss how those specifications would fit with the safety needs of an Electrical Impedance Tomograph. Would it be useful for analog data isolation? Digital isolation? At what transmission rates?

6.5 Find the specifications for any DC-to-DC converter. Would it pass the isolation requirements in this chapter?

7

Interfacing and Computers

Amit Patel

The electrical impedance tomography technique requires a computer system, which can quickly collect the voltage and current data and use these data to calculate the resistivity distribution in the region of interest. The computer controls the hardware for the data collection, reconstructs the image using numerical methods and displays the final image on the screen.

7.1 COMPUTER REQUIREMENTS

The computational speed of the computer determines the time to produce the final image. Most groups working in electrical impedance tomography use a personal computer. A large number of mathematical manipulations is required to process large matrices to reconstruct the image of resistivity distribution. In three-dimensional imaging, much faster computers with larger storage capacity will be required.

7.1.1 Computer speed

With the exception of the backprojection between equipotential lines method, most reconstruction algorithms described in Chapter 10 require much computation. In particular, the modified Newton–Raphson method requires the largest amount of computation compared to other algorithms (see Chapters 10 and 11). Even though modern personal computers use a clock faster than 30 MHz, one of the main difficulties in increasing the spatial resolution of the image is the fact that these computers are not fast enough to perform the image reconstruction in a reasonable amount of computation time.

Recently some groups have used a remote supercomputer (Cray X-MP) for image reconstruction. Also the use of parallel computation is being considered to increase the speed of computation (see Chapter 11).

7.1.2 Storage requirement

In general, the storage requirement of the computer increases with the number of electrodes used, the number of independent measurements obtained, the data collection method, and the length and complexity of the image reconstruction algorithm. However, in most cases, the amount of storage required for the reconstruction algorithm and postprocessing dominates the others.

The total storage requirement is primarily the sum of the storage requirement for data-collection, image reconstruction and image display. However, it is highly dependent on the reconstruction algorithm used. For the same reconstruction algorithm, it varies depending on the detail of the numerical implementation. We will discuss the storage requirement again in Chapter 11.

7.1.3 Computers being used

Yorkey *et al* (1987a) and Liu *et al* (1988) implemented their programs and display on an IBM PC/AT personal computer. Kim and Woo (1987) used an Intel 80286 microprocessor with a 80287 floating point coprocessor for control and image reconstruction and an Intel 80186 microprocessor display board for display. They also used a remote IBM 4341 computer for faster image reconstruction. Murphy *et al* (1987) used a TMS 9995 microprocessor system for data collection and an IBM PC/AT personal computer for image reconstruction and display. Most EIT systems developed so far use a personal computer such as IBM PC/XT or AT for both data acquisition and image reconstruction.

The 32-electrode adaptive EIT system developed by the Wisconsin group uses a Macintosh II for data collection, image reconstruction and display. It has a 16 MHz Motorola 68020 processor with a 68881 floating point coprocessor. It has 8 Mbyte of RAM and 80 Mbyte of hard disk.

The Rensselaer group uses an IBM PC/AT for data collection. They use one of the following computers for image reconstruction: Sun 3/60 workstation, Sun 4/280, IBM 3081-D or Cray X-MP/48. These computers are accessed through a computer network. However, until now, most of the computers used in EIT have been small and inexpensive.

7.2 DIGITAL CONTROL AND DATA COLLECTION SPEED

Figure 1.5 shows how the various stages from the current generation through the display are controlled by a computer. The computer also has a matrix decoder, which collects and later does the computing (not shown in figure 1.5). The oscillator generates an AC signal. Figure 7.1 shows the control scheme used by the Rensselaer group. The magnitude of the AC in the current generators is controlled by a multiplying digital-to-analog converter (DAC) (for certain data collection methods, the magnitude of the peak current is fixed). For a 12-bit DAC, the amplitude can be set at $2^{12} = 1024$ levels. The digital I/O port of a computer sequentially selects a DAC through the address demultiplexer and sets the amplitude of the current generator. Voltage is measured at the voltage electrodes by connecting them to a precision voltmeter. The measured voltages are digitized by an analog-to-digital converter (ADC). Thus the computer controls the current and voltage data collection by programming the I/O port. The control in the Sheffield data collection is done by the hardware shown in figure 7.2.

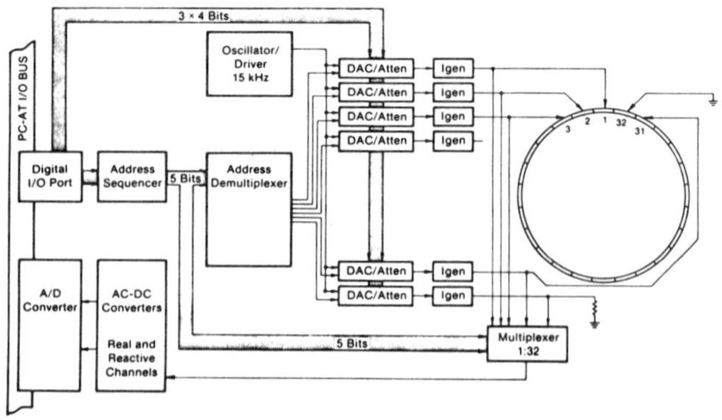

Figure 7.1 The control circuit of an EIT system with gain-controlled current generators (Newell et al 1988).

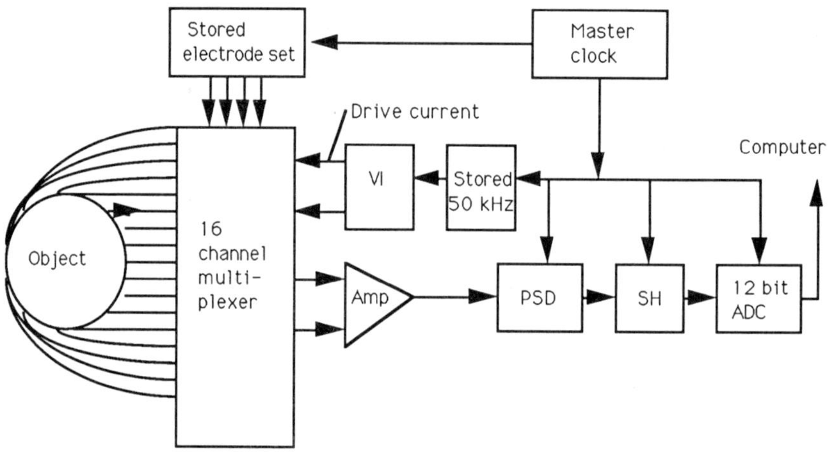

Figure 7.2 The Sheffield data collection system.

A precision voltmeter includes amplifiers, demodulator and low-pass filter. The amplifier amplifies the measured voltage up to a required range after which the data are demodulated. The demodulator should have a fast settling time, to enable fast data acquisition. A higher-order low-pass filter is used for ripple reduction. The ADC should have a sufficient number of bits to ensure low quantization noise in comparison with the dynamic range of the signal. A 12 bit ADC should yield acceptable accuracy. The digitized data are then stored and the resistivity distribution is obtained by implementing numerical methods. The reconstructed image is ultimately displayed on the display screen (usually a color monitor) of the computer. In certain medical and geophysical applications, described in Chapter 13 and Chapter 14, where a portable system is required, a small computer controls the data collection and the collected data are then downloaded into a mainframe computer for image reconstruction and display.

A current-injecting and voltage-measurement cycle includes digital control delay and the settling times of DAC, low-pass filter and ADC. Of all these delays, the settling time of the low-pass filter is the longest. Nowicki *et al* designed a fourth-order Bessel filter whose settling time is 800 μs. Chapter 8 describes the number of measurements each data collection method takes. For an E-electrode system, the number of independent measurements is $E(E-1)/2$, or 496 for a 32-electrode system. Thus the maximal data collection time is 398 ms.

7.3 DISPLAY CAPABILITIES

Once the resistivity distribution is obtained, it is displayed on the screen. It can be displayed on a color monitor, where different colors on the screen correspond to different resistivity values. The Sheffield and Rensselaer groups use an IBM PC/XT or AT with a color monitor for image display. Kim and Woo (1987) use an Intel 80186 as a graphics display processor with a color monitor. The Wisconsin group uses a Macintosh II with a color monitor.

Using a 8 bit video board and color monitor, the current Macintosh II can display 256 colors including 256 different gray levels selected out of about 16 million colors. Although 24 or 32 bit video board and monitors have been developed recently, 256 colors are usually enough for EIT imaging since the resistivity resolution of the reconstructed image does not exceed the 8 bit resolution.

The Macintosh II can also print color images using the ImageWriter printer with a color ribbon (8 colors). Recently, new color printers which can print 256 colors in high resolution have been developed but they are expensive. A Polaroid camera can be used to obtain an image of high resolution, but its high operating cost precludes its use for ordinary applications.

Another common way of displaying and printing images is by using a pattern of black dots, where a range of resistivity is represented by the number of dots per specific region. Figure 7.3 shows that different squares represent different resistivity zones. Each pattern is defined as the number of black dots in a square of 8×8 pixels. By increasing the number of dots from 0 to 63, there are 64 different patterns.

Yorkey *et al* (1987a) and Liu *et al* (1988) used a hatched pattern for the display of the resistivity image. Different hatch patterns represent different resistivity zones.

More sophisticated techniques would be required to display a three-dimensional resistivity distribution. An orthogonal contour plot can be used to display a three-dimensional image. The display can include provision for zooming the image in and out. Multiple windows are useful for the comparison of two or more images.

7.4 STUDY QUESTIONS

7.1 Calculate the number of ports required to control 32 electrodes, 12 bit current sources and describe how the control is accomplished.

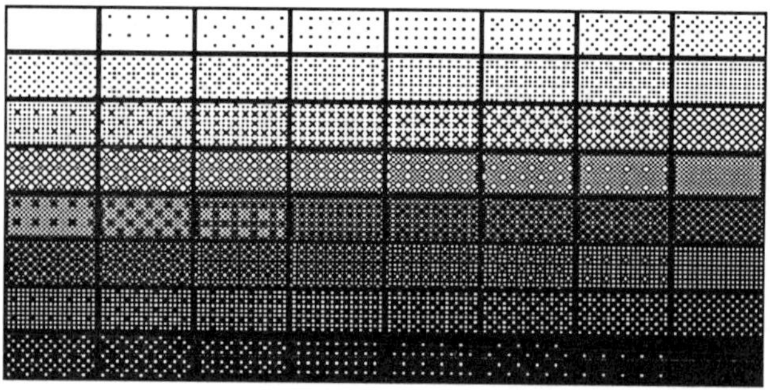

Figure 7.3 In 64 different zones, an increasing number of dots per zone indicates an increasing resistivity.

7.2 Sketch the detail for current-injecting switches and voltage-measuring switches and describe the requirement for each position.
7.3 Sketch the timing diagram for a 32-electrode control system. Label significant times.
7.4 Draw the flowchart for a program that will acquire one frame of data.
7.5 List likely computers for EIT and their advantages and disadvantages.

8

Data Collection Methods

Amit Patel

The goal of electrical impedance tomography is to obtain the resistivity distribution at all points in the plane (or volume) of interest. The resistivity distribution can be obtained by injecting current through the cross section and measuring the voltages at the surface of the cross section between different pairs of electrodes. There are numerous ways in which the current-injecting electrodes are chosen. This chapter describes various methods by which the current is injected and the voltages measured. Once all the current and voltage data are collected at the periphery, the resistivity distribution can be reconstructed by the numerical methods described in Chapter 10. The performance of these data collection methods are described in terms of sensitivity and distinguishability, which are defined in Chapter 12.

8.1 INTRODUCTION

Early systems used the two-electrode method. The voltages were measured from the same electrodes through which the current was injected. The principal source of error in this measuring system was the voltage drop across the skin contact impedance. Thus, some systems replaced the two-electrode data collection method with a four-electrode data collection method. Then the current is injected through some electrodes and the voltage recorded through different electrodes. This method minimizes error in voltage measurement due to the skin contact impedances. In spite of the shortcomings of the two-electrode method over the four-electrode method, it is used for its simplicity in geophysical applications, where accuracy in measurement of the resistivity distribution is not essential.

Lytle and Dines (1978) applied to all electrodes stepped voltages that would produce a uniform current distribution in a homogeneous media. In a nonhomogeneous media, the currents become nonuniform. They measured the resulting currents at all electrodes and repeated the procedure from several angular directions. Kim and Woo (1987) presented a very flexible data collection system, where each of 125 electrodes is programmed separately and various pairs of voltage-injecting and current-measuring electrodes can be selected, to obtain a variety of current distributions. Here 125 electrodes were arranged in five different columns and each column contained 25 electrodes, all placed in a single plane. This method was used for frontal imaging.

Tasto and Schomberg (1978) obtained the voltage–current data points by placing electrodes of different dimensions, insulated from each other, on the opposite sides of a tank filled with saline. The object was placed inside the tank. The front of the tank consisted of 20 metallic electrodes. The rear was completely covered with a large metallic electrode. All the small electrodes were connected via current meters of negligible internal resistance to a low-frequency AC source. The large electrode was connected to the other pole of the source. All small electrodes had equal potential due to the very low resistance of the current meters. The current was measured for each small electrode and was used to determine the resistance of the current path passing from each small electrode to the large electrode.

Sections 8.2 through 8.7 describe the commonly used data collection methods in two-dimensional imaging. We evaluate each method for its current sensitivity. Section 8.8 describes the data collection methods used in three-dimensional imaging. Section 8.9 compares the different data collection methods described in the chapter.

8.2 NEIGHBORING METHOD

Brown and Seagar (1985, 1987) used the neighboring method of data collection. They applied the current through two neighboring electrodes and measured the voltage from all other successive pairs of adjacent electrodes in this four-electrode method. Figure 8.1 shows a data collection system for 16 equally spaced electrodes used for a circular cross section, where the current is applied through electrode pair 1–2. The current flows throughout the circular cross section, with its intensity maximal at the periphery near the current-injecting electrodes and diminishing rapidly towards the opposite side. Figure 8.1 shows the equipotential lines, and the shaded portion between those that terminate on electrodes 6–7 represents the resistivity zone for these electrodes. The voltages are measured between the electrode pairs 3–4, 4–5, 5–6, ... , and 15–16. All 13 voltage measurements are independent. They changed the current-driving pair to 2–3, and measured the voltages similarly between 13 pairs of adjacent electrodes. They rotated the current pair through 3–4, 4–5, ... , 16–1 and for each pair, measured the entire set of the voltages between neighboring electrodes. Thus for a 16-electrode system, they obtained $16 \times 13 = 208$ voltage measurements. However, not all of these data points are independent, since the reversal of voltage and current electrode pairs would give an identical value of the measured resistivity. Thus, because of this reciprocity, only 104 independent measurements are obtained for the above 16-electrode system.

The neighboring method of data collection has a very nonuniform current distribution. Most of the current travels near the peripheral electrodes and hence good sensitivity is obtained at the periphery. This method does not yield good sensitivity at the center because the current density is low there.

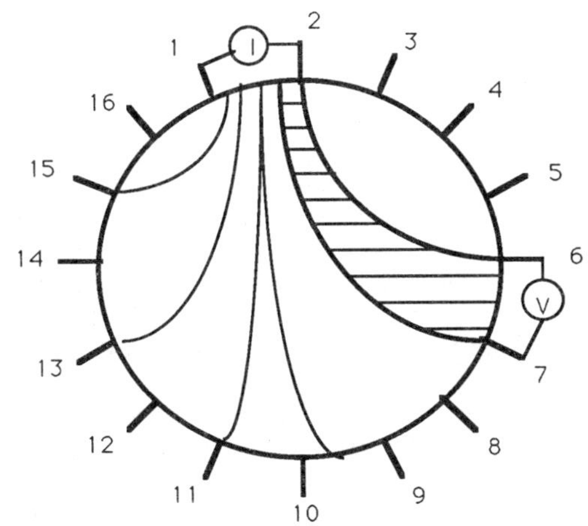

Figure 8.1 In the neighboring method, equipotential lines are formed in a homogeneous medium. Currents injected through neighboring electrodes and voltages measured between adjacent pairs of electrodes.

8.2.1 The Sheffield data collection system

The Sheffield data collection system uses the neighboring method of data collection. Figure 7.2 shows the system. The master clock digitally generates a 51 kHz sinusoidal waveform, which is applied to the voltage to current converter to give an output sinusoidal current of 5 mA peak. The current is applied to a neighboring pair of electrodes and the voltage pairs are selected by addressing the multiplexers. The EPROM addresses the multiplexers and selects a new data set every 79 ms. The voltages are rapidly collected and are sent for further processing (described in Chapter 5) before the current and voltage values are used for reconstruction of the image. If voltages were measured from all 16 electrode pairs, the number of independent measurements would be $E(E-1)/2 = 120$, however, the Sheffield data collection system collects only 104 independent data points. This is because the voltage output from the current electrode pair is not used to reduce the error due to skin contact impedance. Hence, for each of the 16 electrode current pairs, 13 voltage readings are taken. In this case, 104 data points are obtained. The maximal voltage is obtained when the current is applied and the voltage recorded between adjacent pairs of noncurrent-carrying electrodes. The minimal voltage is obtained when the current pair and the voltage pair are on the opposite sides of the cross section (about 2.5% of the maximal voltage). The system sends about ten data sets every second to the computer for reconstruction. The Sheffield group uses a very fast reconstruction algorithm and has the fastest complete system. The spatial resolution of the image obtained is poor, due to the reconstruction algorithm and will be discussed further in Chapter 10.

8.3 CROSS METHOD

Hua *et al* (1987) used the cross method of data collection, where the currents are injected between a pair of electrodes separated by large dimensions. Compared to the neighboring method, the current is more uniformly distributed. Figure 8.2 shows the data collection system. To collect the data set, they made electrode 0 the current-reference electrode and electrode 1 the voltage-reference electrode. They then applied current successively to electrodes 2, 4, ... ,14 and for each current pair measured the voltage with respect to the voltage reference at each electrode except the current electrodes. They then changed the current reference to 3 and the voltage reference to 2 and applied currents through electrodes 5, 7, ... ,15 and 1. They repeated the above procedure for voltage measurement. For each pair of current electrodes 13 voltage measurements were obtained, and 7 different current electrode pairs were selected to give $7 \times 13 = 91$ data points. Another 91 data points could be obtained by changing the voltage and current reference. Thus a 16-electrode system yields a maximum of 182 data points, out of which only 104 are independent measurements. The cross method does not have as good a sensitivity in the periphery as the neighboring method, but, has better matrix conditioning and sensitivity over the entire region.

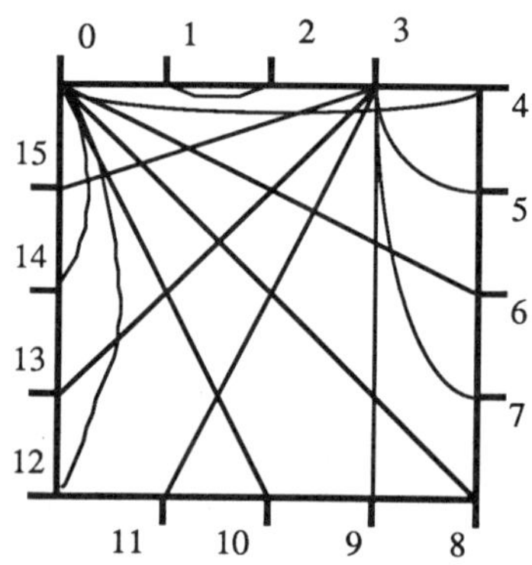

Figure 8.2 In the cross method, current electrodes are separated by large dimensions.

8.4 OPPOSITE METHOD

Hua *et al* (1987) used the opposite method (or 180° method) of data collection. Figure 8.3 shows that current was injected through diametrically opposed electrodes. The voltage reference electrode was adjacent to the current-injecting electrode. For a particular pair of current-injecting electrodes, the voltages were measured with respect to the reference at all the electrodes, except the current-injecting electrodes. To obtain the next set of data, they switched the current to the next pair of opposite electrodes in the clockwise direction. The voltage reference was also changed accordingly, and the voltages were similarly measured with respect to the new reference. The entire image set was obtained by switching the oppositely placed current electrodes through 180°, and the voltages measured for each pair of current electrodes with respect to the reference electrode. For 16 electrodes, this method of data collection gives $8 \times 13 = 104$ data points, with some being redundant. This method has more uniform current density and hence good sensitivity.

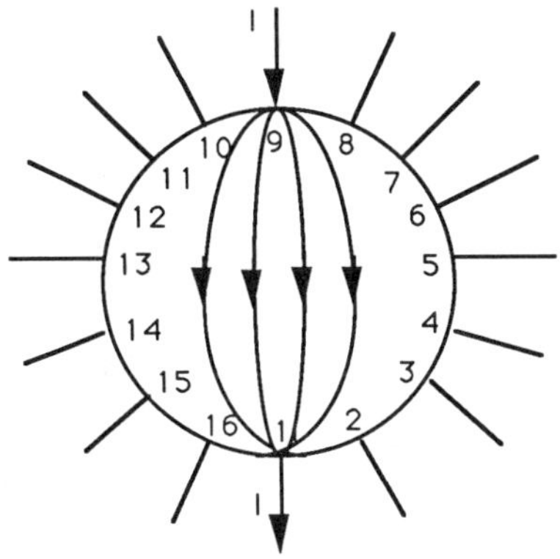

Figure 8.3 In the opposite method, current is injected through diametrically opposed electrodes.

8.5 MULTIREFERENCE METHOD

The data collection methods considered so far use a pair of electrodes through which a single current of constant magnitude is injected, and the voltages are measured across two other electrodes. All the other electrodes are open circuited. Hua *et al* (1987) used the multireference method of data collection, in which they varied the current amplitude in each of many current sources, from 0 to 5 mA. Figure 8.4 shows that for a system with 16 equally spaced electrodes, currents flow through 15 electrodes simultaneously and are collected by the one remaining electrode, which is grounded. Electrode 1 was initially grounded and they injected current through electrodes 2 through 16 simultaneously. They measured the voltages across each of the electrodes 2 through 16 with respect to the reference. They then changed the reference to electrode 2, and injected the current through the remaining 15 electrodes. They measured all the voltages with respect to the new reference. Thus, by varying the reference through one cycle and measuring the voltages and current for each different reference, they obtained a complete data set. For a 16-electrode system, they obtained a total of 240 data points, out of which 120 were independent. To reduce the data collection time and obtain only the independent measurement, approximately eight reference electrodes were used. The current flows through all the electrodes simultaneously, so the error due to the skin contact impedance is reduced, if it is assumed to be constant throughout the periphery. In practice, it is not constant, hence the multireference method of data collection introduces error due to skin contact impedance. For a nonhomogeneous medium of circular cross section, a somewhat uniform current distribution can be obtained by suitable selection of the amplitude of current through the current-injecting electrodes. Due to the somewhat uniform current distribution, this method gives good sensitivity.

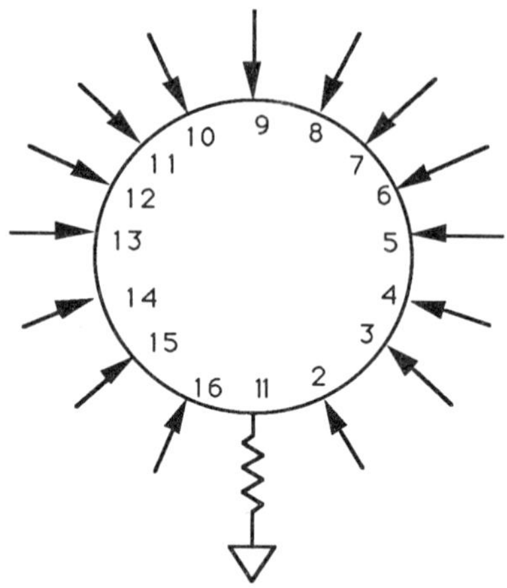

Figure 8.4 In the multireference method, current simultaneously injected through all other electrodes is collected by a single reference electrode.

8.6 ADAPTIVE METHOD

Gisser *et al* (1987) proposed the adaptive method of data collection, where almost any desired current distribution can be obtained by injecting current of appropriate magnitude through all the electrodes simultaneously. This method is also called the optimal current method. Here each electrode can provide output from –5 to +5 mA. The currents flow through all the electrodes simultaneously, which yields voltages obtained with respect to a single grounded electrode. The sensitivity in the desired zone is measured and an algorithm keeps changing the current, until the optimal current is obtained. For a 16-electrode system, 16 current sources are required, which yields a total of 120 independent data points. Figure 8.5 shows that for a homogeneous resistivity distribution, the amplitude of the current in the electrodes follows a cosine curve, to give a perfectly uniform current distribution. This method gives the best distinguishability and is the most versatile method of data collection. In maximizing distinguishability, an interactive experimental process must be pursued to approximate a 'best' current j to distinguish between σ_0 and σ_1. The algorithm for obtaining the 'best' current is described below (Gisser *et al* 1987).

(1) Guess a current density $j_0(\theta)$ for which

$$\int_0^{2\pi} j_0(\theta)d\theta = 0$$

and $|j_0| = 1$. Set $k = 0$.

(2) Measure the voltage $V_k^1(\theta) = R(\sigma_1)j_k(\theta)$ that results from applying $j_k(\theta)$ to the body whose conductivity is σ_1.

(3) Compute the voltage $V_k^0(\theta) = R(\sigma_0)j_k(\theta)$ that would result from applying $j_k(\theta)$ to a body with conductivity σ_0.

(4) Compute the next estimate, $j_{k+1}(\theta)$, to the 'best' current to distinguish σ_0 from σ_1 by $V_k^1(\theta) - V_k^0(\theta)$.

$$j_{k+1}(\theta) = |V_k^1(\theta) - V_k^0(\theta)|.$$

(5) If the changes in j_k are less than the measurement precision ε, i.e., $|j_{k+1} - j_k| < \varepsilon$ stop, otherwise increment k and go to step 2.

Using the methods described above, Gisser *et al* (1987) showed that after five iterations ($k = 5$), 'best' current values converged rapidly toward their theoretically calculated values at $k \approx \infty$.

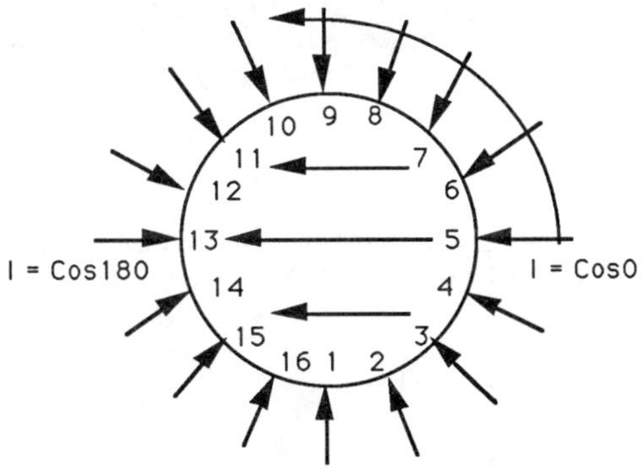

Figure 8.5 In the adaptive method, cosine variation of the amplitude of the current source yields a uniform distribution of current streamlines in a homogeneous medium.

8.7 LINEAR ARRAY

The data collection methods considered so far had electrodes placed all around the cross section. It is not always possible to surround the region of interest with the electrodes, especially in geological applications. Powell *et al* (1985, 1987) used a linear array of electrodes on the top of the surface. They applied a constant current source between two of the electrodes, and measured the voltage between all the adjacent pairs of electrodes, except the current-injecting electrodes. Figure 8.6 shows the equipotential lines for the current injected through a pair of electrodes. The voltage was measured across two intermediate electrodes. An equally spaced 16-electrode system yielded 104 independent data points. The linear array method of data collection has certain disadvantages over the encircling array of electrodes. The current distribution is not specified in a region and the current density is high only in the periphery. Since the current density reduces considerably at a region away from the array, the resolution and sensitivity are very poor away from the array. Figure 8.7 shows that the peak amplitude of the image decreases with distance from the plane of array. The curve shows that the linear array will not detect objects deeper than half an array length. The voltage measured by the linear array method has a greater variation, and thus the signal-processing circuit is more complicated than that in the encircling array method. Since the current spreads out in all three directions, it is difficult to image one particular plane. The linear array method has advantages because it is easy to remove the electrodes. A linear array can give very good spatial resolution near the surface.

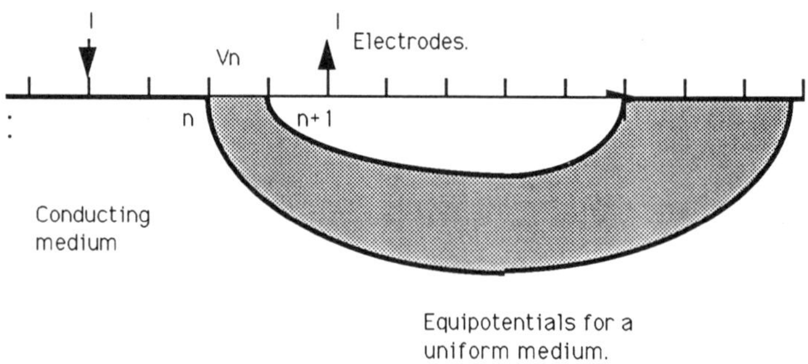

Figure 8.6 In the linear array, equipotential lines are formed in a homogeneous medium. Voltages are measured between adjacent electrodes.

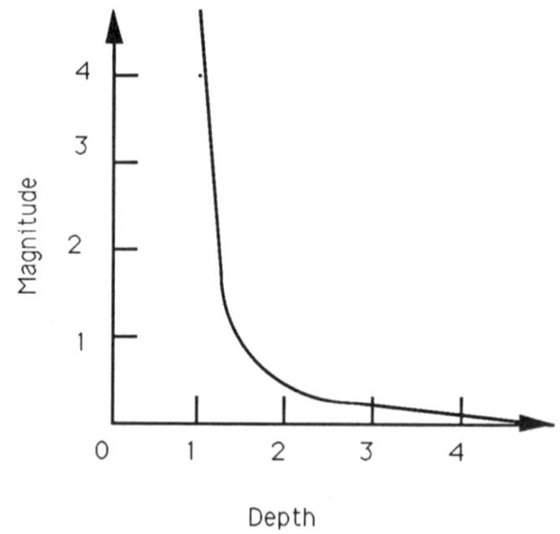

Figure 8.7 The magnitude of the peak amplitude of the image (on an arbitrary linear scale) decreases with depth of the object from a linear array in units equal to electrode spacing.

8.8 THREE-DIMENSIONAL IMAGING

In the imaging considered so far, we assumed that the current was restricted in a single plane. In reality, the current flux spreads out in all three dimensions. The voltage developed by the injected current depends upon the resistivity distribution of the three-dimensional object. Hence, if we put additional electrodes above and below the cross section of interest, we can obtain a three-dimensional resistivity distribution. Figure 8.8 shows that we might inject current through different layers of electrode arrays. Then the current density in the intermediate layers is the superposition of the current density due to each current-injecting array of electrodes. This should yield better three-dimensional imaging.

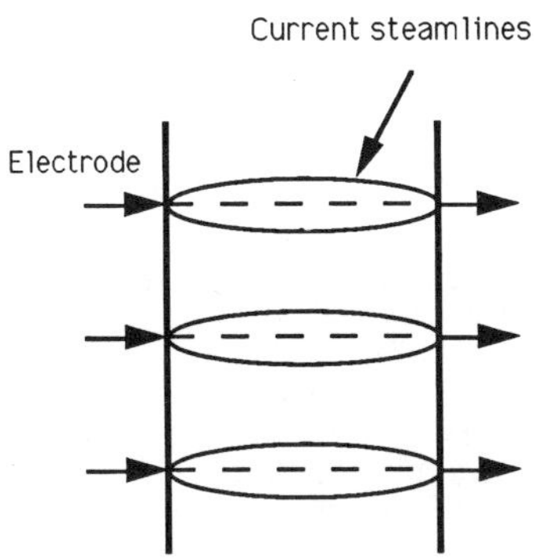

Figure 8.8 A multiple array current-injecting electrode can be used to obtain resistivity distribution in three dimensions.

Because the current flow is not confined to a plane, we require a data collection system which collects data from different planes. The data collection system has electrodes located at the periphery of each different plane for injecting currents and measuring voltages. We obtain the complete measurement data set by injecting current through an electrode pair, and measuring differential voltages between other electrode pairs.

Liu *et al* (1988) suggested a diagonal data collection method for three-dimensional imaging. Figure 8.9 shows a three-dimensional array of current-supplying and voltage-measuring electrodes. It has eight electrodes in each of four different levels, which divides the entire model into three transverse volume layers. They applied current through a pair of neighboring diagonal electrodes and measured the differential voltages from the successive diagonal electrodes placed in the same transverse layer. Then they moved the current-injecting pair of electrodes in the same plane and obtained another set of data. Once they obtained all the current–voltage data from one layer, they applied the current-injecting electrodes to another layer. The complete data set consisted of current–voltage measurements for all three layers. The diagonal method gave 84 independent data points for a 24-electrode system for three transverse layers. Liu *et al* (1988) reported that the diagonal method is better than the neighboring method in most cases. In a special case, when the object had resistivity variation only in two directions, the neighboring method of data collection resulted in a better reconstructed image.

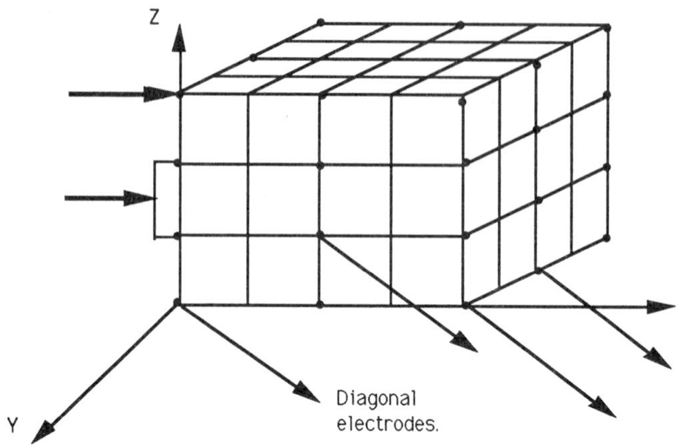

Figure 8.9 In the diagonal method, voltages are measured across the two electrodes placed diagonally on the same transverse plane.

Wexler *et al* (1985) suggested a method of data collection for subsurface imaging. Figure 8.10 shows a three-dimensional cubic grid of nodes defined over the region of interest. They placed electrodes on the nodes on top of the surface. They injected current from an electrode pair, and took voltage measurements from different pairs of electrodes. This method gave useful resistivity information for objects close to the surface.

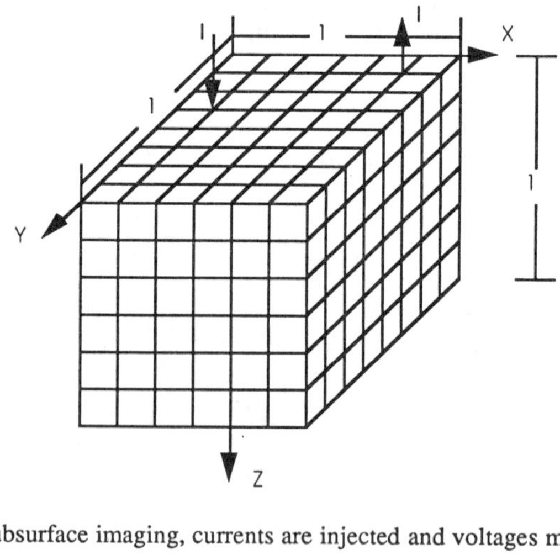

Figure 8.10 For subsurface imaging, currents are injected and voltages measured only from the top surface.

Goble and Isaacson (1989) extended the adaptive method in two dimensions into three dimensions. They used the method of Gisser *et al* to derive the three-dimensional 'best currents' for a three-dimensional electrode layout. They then injected these current patterns into the object simultaneously through all the electrodes and measured the voltages from them. Goble and Isaacson showed that these currents had better distinguishability than injecting current in one plane.

Ider *et al* (1989) developed an algorithm for compensating for three-dimensional effects in EIT. If electrodes are placed around a single plane only, and in the absence of any additional information regarding the three-dimensional impedance distribution, we may proceed by making some assumptions. It has been shown that for cylindrical object with axial uniformity in impedance, the three-dimensional forward solution can be decomposed into a series of 20 forward solutions by making use of Fourier expansions of boundary conditions and the field distribution in the axial direction. This method can be used to obtain the reference needed by the backprojection method of reconstruction and thus may be applied to objects with relatively uniform axial impedance distribution (arms and legs).

8.9 COMPARISION OF DATA COLLECTION METHODS

Hua *et al* (1987) simulated measurement error by superimposing random noise on the theoretical measured data. Figure 8.11 shows the reconstruction error for different added noise levels for different data collection methods. The reconstruction was done using the Newton–Raphson method and the reconstruction error was defined as the difference between the true resistivity value and the theoretically estimated resistivity value. Figure 8.12 compares the different data collection methods in terms of their performance.

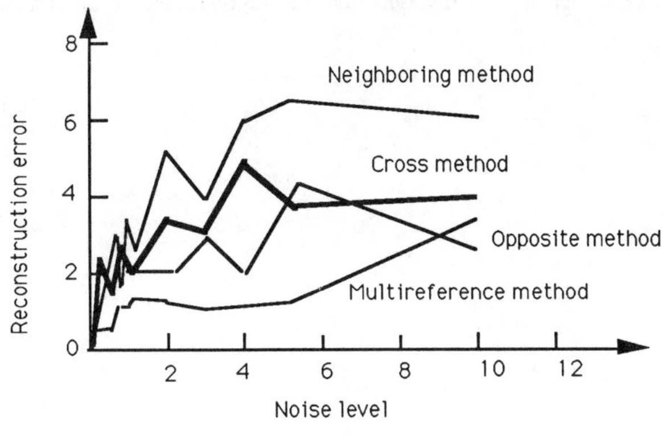

Figure 8.11 When noise is added, the multireference method yields the lowest error.

Data collection method	Current distribution in the cross section	Spatial resolution and distinguishability
Neighboring method	Very poor at the center	Poor
Cross method	Uniform	Good
Opposite method	Uniform	Good
Multireference method	Very uniform	Very good
Adaptive method	Very uniform	Very good
Linear array	High only near the surface	Good for depth up to 2 electrode spacing

Figure 8.12 Comparison of the different data collection methods for a 16-electrode system.

8.10 STUDY QUESTIONS

8.1 For the neighboring method, describe the data collection method and sketch a flow chart.

8.2 For the cross method, describe the data collection method to obtain a complete data set.

8.3 For the adaptive method, describe the data collection method to obtain a complete data set.

8.4 Explain the advantages and disadvantages of the multireference data collection method, as compared to the adaptive method.

8.5 For a two-dimensional linear array of eight electrodes, sketch the equipotentials for a uniform medium. Sketch the current flux lines.

8.6 For a three-dimensional array, describe the diagonal method of data collection.

9

Data Collection Errors

Mark Heimbach

This chapter describes properties and limitations of electronic instrumentation and also measurement error characteristics of an electrical impedance tomography (EIT) system. Although many sources of error exist in EIT imaging, many are negligible in a practical system and can be ignored. However, specific sources of error are dependent on a variety of factors including imaging techniques, number of electrodes, reconstruction algorithms and the visibility of the object to be imaged. We desire to minimize the error in resistivity in EIT. Thus we must understand the significance of data collection errors as caused by various components of the EIT system. In this way we can design effective imaging systems to produce the needed image quality for a given application.

9.1 OSCILLATOR AMPLITUDE JITTER

Oscillator amplitude jitter is the change of the output signal amplitude caused by noise from various sources. The presence of amplitude jitter degrades the impedance measurements in EIT systems, becoming particularly prominent under conditions where signal averaging can not be performed. One source of noise is created by random fluctuations in electronic junctions. Transient surges in line voltage can cause random fluctuations in the output amplitude of the oscillator signal.

We tested several oscillators for their amplitude stability at room temperature. An LM7805 voltage regulator was connected at the input of each oscillator power supply to minimize fluctuations from line voltage. At the operating frequency of 50 kHz, the LM7805 provided a rejection ratio of 80 dB. The oscillator output was then rectified and passed through a low-pass filter where the output signal was measured with a storage oscilloscope (see figure 9.1). The low-pass filter had a corner frequency of 24.4 Hz in order to attenuate by a factor of $1/2^{12}$ the ripple frequencies at 100 kHz to achieve 12 bit accuracy. This filter had a time constant of $\tau = 1/[2\pi(24.4)] = 6.5$ ms. After each switching we must wait 10τ so the error diminishes by a factor of $1/2^{12}$. $10\tau = 10(6.5 \text{ ms}) = 65$ ms. Thus we sampled every 70 ms.

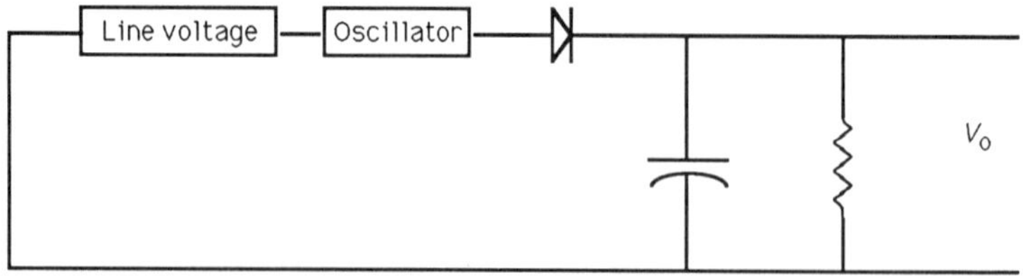

Figure 9.1 To measure oscillator jitter, output must be rectified and filtered.

Figure 9.2 shows a FET-stabilized Wien-bridge oscillator designed specifically for high-amplitude stability (Van der Walt 1981). This has less than 0.01% distortion over a temperature range from 0 to 40°C. The output voltage of the oscillator is full-wave rectified and compared with a reference voltage. The difference between these voltages is then integrated and filtered. This signal is then fed to the gate of a FET which varies the oscillator feedback resistance to maintain a constant amplitude.

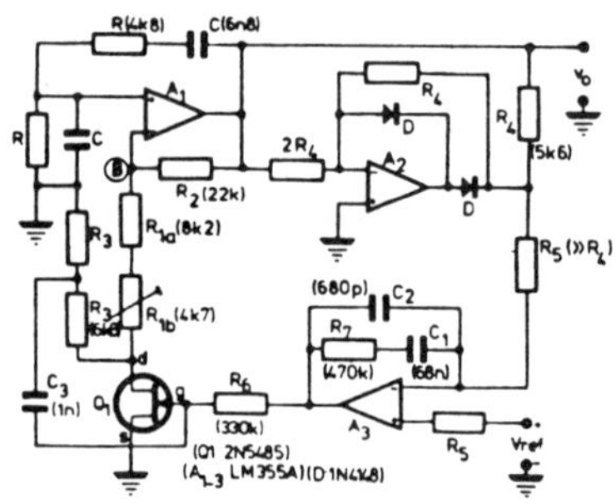

Figure 9.2 The output of this Wien-Bridge oscillator is compared to a reference to permit feedback stabilization using FET impedance.

The second oscillator tested was an integrated circuit (XR-2206). Tests made on the XR-2206 produced a harmonic distortion of 0.1%. We were not interested in harmonic distortion as much as amplitude stability and conducted tests to measure this amplitude jitter. For the Wien-bridge oscillator, jitter was measured to be 1.68 mV, while the XR-2206 produced a more stable signal with a jitter of 0.36 mV. The XR-2206 oscillator jitter compared closely with the $1/2^{12}$ error for a 12 bit system.

9.2 ELECTRODE LOCATION ERROR

In EIT imaging systems, a measured data set is compared with a homogeneous calculated data set to measure resistivity differences from a uniform reference. However, to obtain this homogeneous data set we must know the exact position of the surface electrodes. Additionally, errors based on imprecise measurements of electrode width contribute to overall errors in the data set.

The magnitude of electrode location error is not only a function of the difference between real and calculated electrode positions, but is also directly related to the magnitude of the gradient of the electric field where the measurement is taken. Figure 9.3 shows that using the cross method, Hu *et al* (1986) measured voltage changes of 2.3%/mm of full scale in positions located near current-generating electrodes. However, these voltage changes decreased significantly to 0.01%/mm of full scale when electrodes were moved to the least sensitive position. These errors were much larger than errors caused by noise, unbalanced constant current sources, and system nonlinearity. In order to minimize these errors, a precise layout of the electrodes in the construction of a physical phantom is needed to within tolerances of 3% to keep the average error less than 1%.

	% of full scale	% of total error
Electrical noise	0.020	0.844
Unbalanced current	0.032	1.351
Nonlinearity	0.007	0.295
Most sensitive electrode change	2.300/mm	97.090
Least sensitive electrode change	0.010/mm	0.422

Figure 9.3 Voltage errors caused by electrode location are much larger than others in EIT. Electrode location error is calculated for 1.0 mm.

Another source of error exists when electrode widths vary from an expected value. Figure 9.4 shows the magnitude of error in voltage measurements when actual electrode widths are larger than an assumed point electrode. Due to varying tissue impedances, voltages at neighboring electrodes will have different potentials. With an increase in electrode surface area, tissue impedance between electrodes decreases allowing unpredicted surface current to flow between electrodes. Yorkey (1986) measured this error using a square physical phantom with four electrodes driven by an oscillator connected to one side while four grounded electrodes were connected to the opposite side. The boundary voltages for the source were 0.72 V while voltages for the supposedly grounded electrodes ranged from 0.27 V to 0.06 V. The reconstructed image had no resemblance to the actual phantom model.

While it is theoretically feasible to precisely measure the position of an array of electrodes around the body, it has not been accomplished in practice. One possible method is to make a rigid mold containing the electrodes and fill it with saline. A rigid circular mold has been built for the breast. However, this is not practical for large sections of the body such as the thorax (Brown and Barber 1987). A fixed linear array of electrodes can be directly pressed into contact with the body. This is useful for imaging objects relatively close to the body surface such as the bladder.

The need for accurate knowledge of electrode locations also disappears if only changes in tissue resistivity are of interest. In dynamic imaging, backprojection of a collected data set is made with an initial data set instead of a

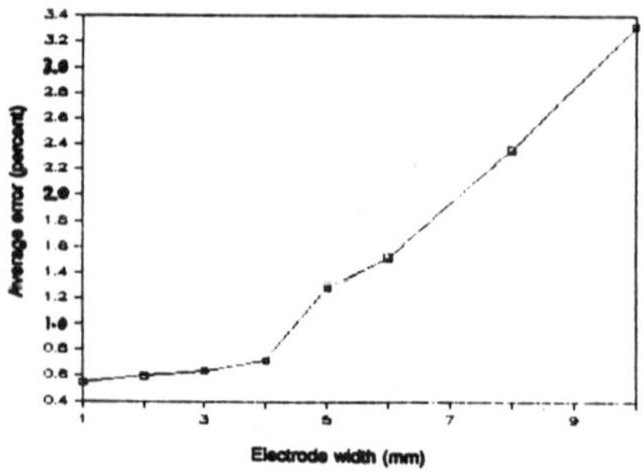

Figure 9.4 Voltage error measurement increases with electrode width in EIT.

homogeneous data set. While the spatial resolution in such systems is poor, the sensitivity to change in resistivity is high.

Barber and Brown (1988b) described a method of determining body shape from multiple impedance measurements. The voltage measured between a pair of electrodes on a body surface when a current is injected between a second pair of electrodes on the surface depends upon the relative positions of the electrodes, the shape of the body surface and the internal impedance distribution. Their method utilizes the fact that a measured voltage is most strongly dependent on the electrode position and the shape of the body surface.

If E electrodes are connected to the body surface, then $E(E - 3)/2$ independent measurements can be made using the neighboring method (Section 8.2). The voltage measured between electrodes (k, l) when current I is injected between electrodes (i, j) is given by

$$V_{ijkl} = I \cdot F(\boldsymbol{r}_i, \boldsymbol{r}_j, \boldsymbol{r}_k, \boldsymbol{r}_l, b(\boldsymbol{r}), c(\boldsymbol{r})) \tag{9.1}$$

where $\boldsymbol{r}_i$ etc are the positions of the electrodes, $b(\boldsymbol{r})$ is a function representing the boundary and $c(\boldsymbol{r})$ is the internal impedance distribution. Since V_{ijkl} is only weakly dependent on $c(\boldsymbol{r})$, this is replaced by a constant C. Similarly since the dependence on $b(\boldsymbol{r})$ is weaker than that on electrode position, this can be combined into a single function F' of the electrode position. Then we obtain

$$V_{ijkl} = I \cdot C \cdot F'(\boldsymbol{r}_i, \boldsymbol{r}_j, \boldsymbol{r}_k, \boldsymbol{r}_l) \tag{9.2}$$

Given the set of measured voltages and a model of the function F', the position vectors $\boldsymbol{r}$ of the E electrodes can be found and hence the boundary obtained. In the absence of an exact model of F', the fact that there are $E(E - 3)/2$ independent measurements and only $2E$ electrode coordinates to compute means that the problem is usefully overdetermined and hence leads to robust solutions for electrode positions.

They suggested the following simple form for F':

$$F'(d) = \frac{1}{d_{ik}{}^n} \tag{9.3}$$

where d_{ik} is the distance between the midpoint between the drive and voltage measurement electrode pairs. A value of n = 3.7 was used. However, no evidence has been produced to show that this form of F' is optimal.

9.3 STRAY CAPACITANCE ERROR

Current sources require cables that lead to the subject. Figure 9.5 shows that the stray capacitance of 100 pF shunts the output of the current source and lowers its output impedance. Cable shields can be driven to minimize this error. Several current sources were tested and the following results were obtained.

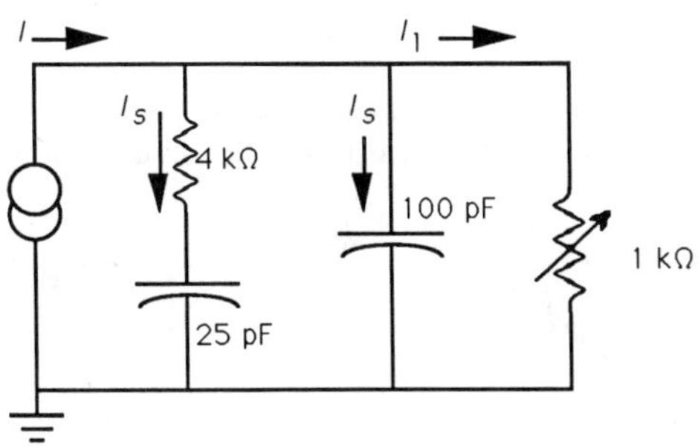

Figure 9.5 Nonideal current source with stray capacitance diverting current away from load.

Figure 9.5 shows a model of a nonideal current source whose output is shunted from the load by a stray capacitance of 100 pF on the cable with a driven shield (see Section 4.5). We tested several current sources and measured output impedances typically in the range of 4 kΩ – j260 kΩ at 50 kHz. When compared to cable capacitances of 100 pF, the current source impedance was found to be negligible (adding a value of 1.06 Ω to the effective shunt impedance caused by the cable alone). This shunt impedance diverts 0.39% of a unity current giving a load current of 1.001 at an angle of 0.9°. When demodulated, such errors are negligible when compared with the accuracy required for a 12 bit system (less than 0.00025). When needed, op amps with gains of 400–600 at 50 kHz can be used to drive shields to further reduce shunt capacitance. For our typical stray capacitance of 100 pF and an op-amp gain of 600, the effective capacitance, in theory, is lowered to 100 pF/600 = 0.167 pF or a shunt impedance of 19.1 MΩ. However, fringing effects at the end of shields and the use of nonideal op amps for shielding allow some stray capacitance to be present. Seagar *et al* (1987) reported that capacitances as low as 1 pF could be achieved in practical experiments. Such shielding can be incorporated in systems using extralong cable networks.

EIT current of 5 mA flowing through skin contact impedance of 200 Ω produces 1 V of common mode voltage V_{cm}. This common mode voltage is attenuated by the skin contact impedance, which is shunted by the stray capacitance of 100 pF of the wire leading to the voltmeter amplifier. The differential amplifier measures the output of two different attenuators and this causes common mode to differential conversion. In order to minimize these effects, cable shields can be driven, or a buffer can be incorporated into the electrode.

9.4 QUANTIZATION ERROR

The measurements obtained for EIT are processed by a computer in order to reconstruct an image. Since all analog values must be converted to digital form to be used by a computer, they must be quantized by partitioning the analog changes of voltages into 4096 discrete ranges. All analog values within a given range are represented by the same digital code. In the A/D conversion process, an ADC yields quantization errors of ±1/2 LSB (least significant bit). Figure 9.6 shows the bit errors for ideal ADC and DAC systems.

For a 12 bit system, this quantization error is 1.26 mV in a 10 V system. Since many other error sources fall well below the 1.26 mV error, the quantization error seems to be the limiting factor in determining the accuracy in EIT.

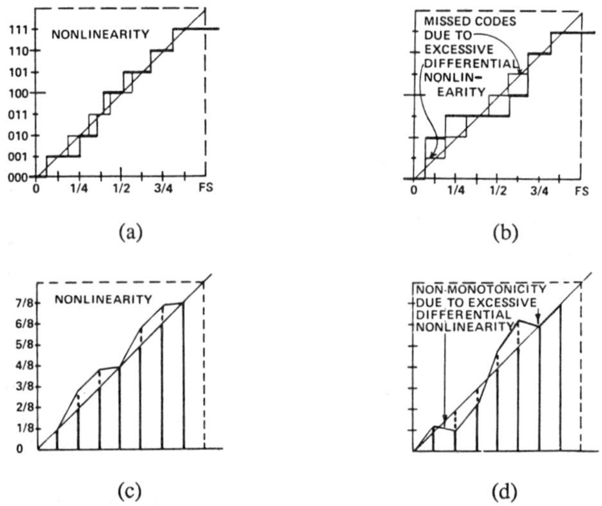

Figure 9.6 Nonlinearity errors for ADCs and DACs. (a) Linearity error in 3 bit ADC. (b) Missed codes in 3 bit ADC. (c) Linearity error in 3 bit DAC. (d) Nonmonotonicity due to excessive differential nonlinearity in 3 bit DAC.

9.5 NONLINEARITY

Any deviation of input–output characteristics from a straight line is nonlinearity. Forms of nonlinearity include saturation, breakdown, dead band (where output is constant until a threshold input value is reached) and hysteresis. The degree of nonlinearity of a component is frequency dependent. Expected sources of nonlinearity in the EIT hardware include the current generator, the demodulator and the ADC. In the ADC conversion process, errors occur due to transition values for each bit change not being all equal or uniformly changing. In systems with large linearity errors, whole bit changes can be missed causing measurable errors in the system. In EIT systems, nonlinear effects are negligible (see figure 9.3).

9.6 NOISE

Ignoring all other sources of error, the best resolution and accuracy of an EIT system can be obtained where the fractional change in voltage may be taken as being equal to the noise (Seagar and Brown 1987). Noise is either random or associated directly with some noise-generating component in the system. Such coherent noise is generated by devices such as power supplies and modulation/demodulation circuits. This noise is small and can be minimized with isolation, shielding and filtering signals at various stages within the system. Most noise is random and arises within the junction of the transistor of the first stage of amplification. The magnitude of error due to noise is typically in the microvolt range and thus is negligible compared to the quantization noise, which is in the millivolt range.

Random noise is a source of error at low frequencies (less than 100 Hz) where electrode noise becomes significant. However, at frequencies in the 50 kHz range this problem is negligible. Movement artifact is a more important source of noise. Where needed, the signal to noise ratio (SNR) can be improved by averaging a number of repetitions to reduce the noise which is generally random in nature. If N repetitions of signal are added, the sum signal has a SNR improved by a factor of $N^{1/2}$.

9.7 CONTACT IMPEDANCE

The electrode-skin contact impedance at 50 kHz is in the range of 200–400 Ω cm^2. This compares with typical tissue impedance of 100 Ω. Figure 9.7 by Yorkey (1986) shows a circuit model for electrode impedances where R_t represents the equivalent model tissue resistance, R_c the electrode contact resistance and R_i the internodal resistance. An additional source of impedance occurs with switch resistance (about 200 Ω) which is known and can be accounted for in the reconstruction algorithm. A problem with contact impedance occurs in that there is no functional relationship between currents measured at electrode sites and voltages across tissues due to unknown and varying contact impedances at each electrode site. These contact impedances are subject to a variation of several hundred ohms depending on the contact area and thickness of the skin. Although electrode contact impedances can be accounted for in reconstruction algorithms, problems occur when different impedances are present at each electrode location. These errors are particularly significant where the measurement of currents is made at current-injection electrodes in two-electrode systems. Using typical values of contact impedance and tissue resistance, 300 Ω and 100 Ω respectively, an input voltage of 50 mV will cause a voltage drop across the tissues of 12.5 mV. However, if the total contact impedance dropped from 300 Ω to 250 Ω, then the voltage across the tissue would be 14.3 mV or an error of 1.79 mV. In conditions where electrode contact impedances vary greatly due to humidity, condition of the skin, etc., these errors would escalate to intolerable levels.

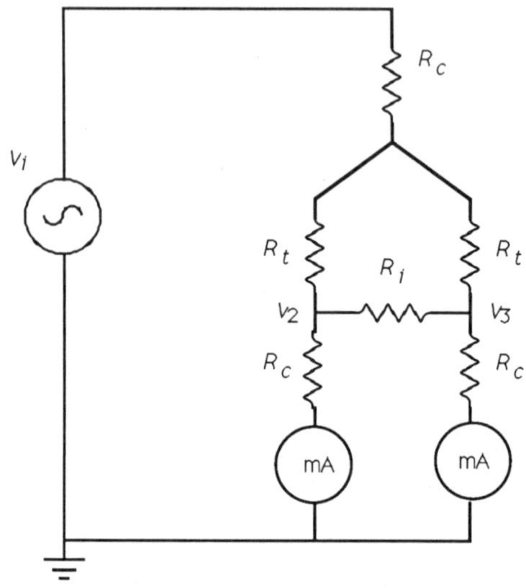

Figure 9.7 Circuit model for contact impedance. A potential between V_2 and V_3 causes unwanted shunt current to flow between electrodes.

Yorkey (1986) proposed the use of voltage clamps to minimize these errors by lowering the apparent electrode contact resistance to 10 Ω. The voltage clamp system requires the addition of an amplifier and electrode for each existing electrode plus digital logic hardware and analog switches. The additional electrode senses the voltage on the phantom and drives the output electrode, clamping the boundary voltage to a desired level. However, contact impedance problems are minimized in four-electrode systems when voltages are measured at sites where current is not injected (Wexler *et al* 1985). With a constant current source, the injected boundary currents are independent of any contact impedances. The measured voltages are also independent of contact impedance for voltage amplifiers with sufficiently high input impedances. Additional hardware such a voltage clamps would therefore not be needed. Using the four-electrode system has both the advantage of minimizing contact impedance errors while simplifying the instrumentation.

The data collection methods such as neighboring method, cross method and opposite method in fact use the four-electrode method. These methods inject current through one pair of current electrodes and measure the voltage on all electrodes except the current electrodes. Data collection methods such as the adaptive method and the multireference method inject current through all the electrodes and measure voltages from all these electrodes. However, Cheng *et al* (1989) showed that the data from these latter methods generate better images than the former methods. This is because the current patterns have better distinguishability.

Hua *et al* (1989) developed a compound electrode system which injects current through an inner electrode and senses voltage from outer electrodes. This system can inject current patterns while minimizing the contact impedance problem in the two-electrode method. Thus it is capable of collecting data with maximal information and a minimal contact impedance problem.

Hua *et al* (1989) developed a FEM model for the contact layer. They imposed two constraints on the model: (1) The electrode is equipotential. (2) The total current is the measured current. They found the element matrix is a function of the product of resistivity and thickness of the contact layer. The FEM model thus described models the shunting and edge effect of the contact layer.

Hua *et al* (1989) incorporated the FEM model for the contact layer into their reconstruction process. They defined the product of resisitivity and thickness of an electrode as a new variable. They treated it the same as the internal resistivity distribution and estimated the contact impedances using the reconstruction algorithms. Different impedances were present at each electrode location. However, due to the constraints of the number of unknowns for a given electrode number, they estimated the average value of these impedances. This method improved the reconstruction accuracy significantly.

9.8 RECIPROCITY ERROR

Rosell *et al* (1989) used the reciprocity theorem to test their parallel data acquisition system using phantoms. The reciprocity theorem says that the voltage measured by a pair of electrodes when current is injected through another pair, should be same as the measured voltage when we interchange the voltage measuring and current-injecting electrode pairs. In practice, these voltages do not coincide and they calculated an average reciprocity error as the square root of the sum of the squares of the differences between reciprocal values, divided by the number of value pairs.

They injected 10 kHz current through a pair of electrodes from 16 total electrodes and measured voltage with 12 bit accuracy. They obtained a reciprocity error of 1.5% using a phantom with sixteen 200 Ω resistors simulating electrode impedance and 1% without the resistors. When they short-circuited any one of the resistors, the error increased up to 2.4%. When the system was applied to a human thorax, they obtained a reciprocity error of 10–20%.

They used the reciprocity error to evaluate the effect of common-mode feedback. They showed that the reciprocity error could be decreased from 65% to 1.2% by using common-mode feedback with a feedback gain of 5 at 10 kHz. The reciprocity error was increased from 1.2% to 1.6% and 1.9% when the feedback gain was 2.5 and 1.7, respectively. They suggested the reciprocity error as a way to estimate measurement errors and reported that they could reconstruct dynamic images using the weighted backprojection algorithm when the reciprocity error was approximately 30%.

9.9 STUDY QUESTIONS

9.1 When testing for amplitude jitter, what time constant should we use in the filter measuring the voltage? Explain.

9.2 Explain why electrode position errors are not a problem in the Sheffield system.

9.3 Explain how you would minimize electrode position errors on human subjects.

9.4 List each location where stray capacitance could cause a problem and the reason why it would cause a problem.

9.5 Calculate the quantization error for a 12 bit system. Compare this with other errors in the system.

9.6 List the expected sources of nonlinearity in EIT.

9.7 Calculate the magnitude of amplifier random noise.

9.8 Calculate the CMRR required for the amplifier.

9.9 Explain how a driven-right-leg circuit would or would not help the CMRR problem.

9.10 Estimate the electrode-skin contact impedance at 50 kHz and compare it with typical tissue impedance.

10

Reconstruction Algorithms

Ping Hua and Eung Je Woo

This chapter presents various reconstruction algorithms used in EIT. It first explains the nature of the reconstruction problem. It then describes the methods of solving the problem, including the equipotential line method, the perturbation method, the double constraint method, the Newton–Raphson method and the compensation theorem method. It also describes the finite element method as the basic tool to implement these reconstruction methods. Finally, the chapter compares the performance of different algorithms.

The chapter makes use of the data acquired by the data collection methods and the hardware described in previous chapters.

10.1 INTRODUCTION

The electric field is governed by Poisson's equation

$$\nabla\cdot\rho^{-1}\nabla V = f \tag{10.1}$$

with boundary conditions

$$V = V_0 \quad \text{on } \partial A \tag{10.2}$$

$$\rho^{-1}\partial V/\partial n = J_0 \quad \text{on } \partial A \tag{10.3}$$

where ρ, V and f are the resistivity, voltage and impressed current source distributions within the region being studied, and ∇ is $i\partial/\partial x + j\partial/\partial y + k\partial/\partial z$, the Poisson operator. V_0 and J_0 are the voltage and current density at the boundary region.

In EIT, we use 50 kHz currents to map the impedance distribution. Since there are no current sources of this frequency within our body, f = 0. Therefore, equation (10.1) becomes

$$\nabla\cdot\rho^{-1}\nabla V = 0. \tag{10.4}$$

For a homogeneous medium, ρ is a constant. Thus for the special case, which is not used, the governing equation can be further degenerated into Laplace's equation.

$$\Delta V = 0 \tag{10.5}$$

where $\Delta = \nabla \cdot \nabla = \partial^2/\partial x^2 + \partial^2/\partial y^2 + \partial^2/\partial z^2$, the Laplace operator.

Using high-frequency current provides electrical safety and small electrode skin contact impedance. Also we do not have to consider low-frequency current generators, such as the heart. This simplifies the problem.

The above relations use x and y coordinates in the two-dimensional case and x, y and z in the three-dimensional case.

10.2 FORWARD VS. INVERSE PROBLEM

10.2.1 Forward problem

Figure 10.1 shows the definition of the forward problem. Given the resistivity distribution with boundary current density and voltage distributions, solve for the internal voltage and current density distributions.

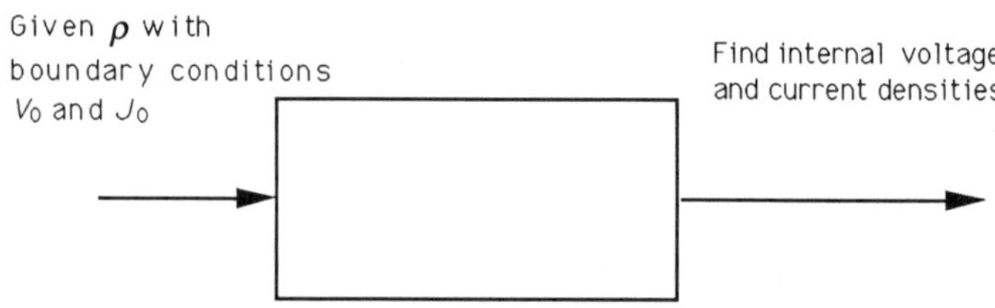
Given ρ with
boundary conditions
V0 and J0
Find internal voltages V
and current densities J

Figure 10.1 The forward problem finds internal voltages and current densities.

10.2.2 Inverse problem

Figure 10.2 shows the definition of the inverse problem. Given the voltage and current density distributions, solve for the resistivity distribution. Generally speaking, the numerical solution of an inverse problem requires iterative solutions of a forward problem.

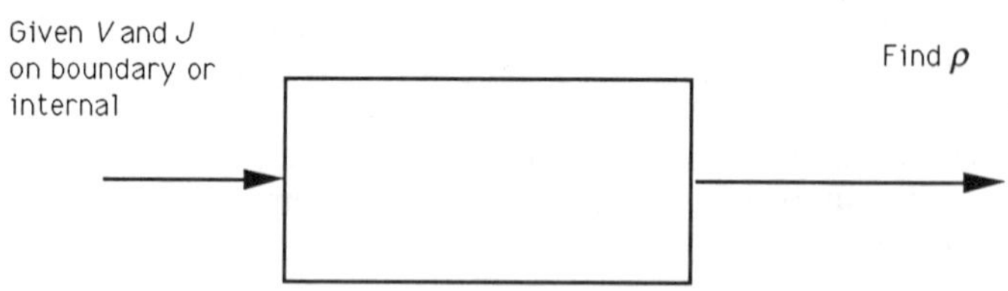

Figure 10.2 The inverse problem finds the resistivity distribution.

10.2.3 Boundary value problem

Figure 10.3 shows the definition of a boundary value problem. Given boundary current density and voltage distributions, solve for the resistivity distribution or voltage or current density distribution.

In EIT, we measure the voltage and current distributions on the electrodes placed at the periphery of a body, and determine the body's internal resistivity distribution. Most people would call this an inverse problem but some people would call this a boundary value problem, which includes solving an inverse problem.

The governing equation (10.4) is a very complicated differential equation, and it is impossible to achieve its general analytic solution. Therefore, a numerical method, namely the finite element method (FEM), is usually employed to derive the solutions.

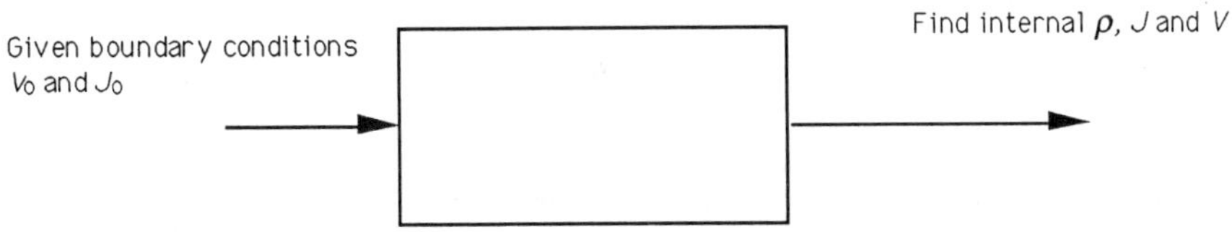

Figure 10.3 A boundary problem uses the inverse problem to find the ρ, V, and J.

10.3 FINITE ELEMENT APPROXIMATION

For the reconstruction of the resistivity image, we need to solve the forward problem. Since we can not analytically solve the forward problem for an arbitrary resistivity distribution, we should use a numerical technique such as the Finite Difference Method (FDM) or Finite Element Method (FEM). It is well known that the FEM is better than the FDM for arbitrary shaped boundaries. In addition, the FEM gives a piecewise approximation to the governing equation (10.4) whereas the FDM gives a pointwise approximation. Therefore, most reconstruction algorithms in EIT use the FEM in solving the forward problem.

In the FEM, we change the calculus problem ($\nabla\rho^{-1}\nabla V = 0$) into the algebraic problem ($\mathbf{Y}\boldsymbol{v} = \boldsymbol{c}$, a linear system of equations), then we solve the linear system of equations using various numerical techniques.

10.3.1 Discretization of the physical medium (mesh generation)

Discretization

First, we divide the domain into a finite number of elements. We usually use triangular or quadrilateral elements in a two-dimensional problem and tetrahedral or hexahedral elements in a three-dimensional problem. In EIT, we assume that the resistivity in each element is homogeneous and isotropic. The discretization process converts the continuous problem into a problem with a finite number of unknowns by expressing the unknown field variables (voltages) in terms of certain interpolation functions within each element. The interpolation functions are defined in terms of the values of the field variables at nodes of the element. Therefore, the nodal values of the field variables become new unknowns and the values of the field variables inside the elements are determined from the nodal values by the interpolation functions. We know that the solution of the FEM converges to the true solution as the element size decreases to zero (Burnett 1987, Huebner and Thornton 1975).

Special consideration for impedance imaging

For a reconstruction algorithm like the modified Newton–Raphson method described in this chapter, the number of elements limits the spatial resolution of the resistivity image. Therefore, in developing the finite element model for EIT, we must consider not only the accuracy of the amplitude of the solution of the forward problem but also the spatial resolution it provides. A fine mesh provides both good accuracy and spatial resolution. However, the design of the mesh is strictly limited by the following relationships.

Number of electrodes, number of independent measurements, and spatial resolution

Let the number of electrodes be E, then the number of independent measurements is $E(E-1)/2$ (Yorkey 1986). Since it is equivalent to the maximal number of equations, the maximal number of resistivity values (unknowns) we can determine is limited by this number. However, in practice, we can only determine a number of resistivity values less than this number due to the nonlinear nature of the problem. Therefore, the spatial resolution of the resistivity image is primarily determined by the number of electrodes used in the EIT system.

Grouping of elements

When a generated mesh contains many elements to provide a good accuracy for the forward problem, we frequently need to constrain some elements by forcing them to have the same resistivity value. This decreases the spatial resolution. Element grouping requires a careful implementation when used with the modified Newton–Raphson reconstruction algorithm. Image reconstruction fails without grouping if the finite element mesh selected contains too many independent elements.

An example of a finite element mesh

Woo *et al* (1988) developed a finite element mesh with efficient global node renumbering schemes. Figure 10.4 shows the model of a circular two-dimensional phantom for a 32-electrode EIT system. This model consists of 389 nodes and 536 triangular or quadrilateral elements. The size of each element was determined so that it could provide 5% spatial resolution for resistivity. We modeled the region around each electrode with 3 elements (2 under each electrode and 1 between pairs of electrodes) resulting in the total of 96 elements in the outermost layer. This permitted solving the forward problem accurately since voltage changes are large in this region. Even though we need many elements in the outside layers for accuracy, we do not usually need high spatial resolution there. Therefore, we constrained the elements in the two or three outermost layers by assigning the same resistivity value to two or four elements since the resistance in this region including the electrode–skin resistance does not change rapidly from region to region. There are 376 resistivity values to be determined by the reconstruction algorithm. Since there are 496 independent measurements from the 32 electrodes, these 376 resistivity values can be determined from the measured voltage data on the surface.

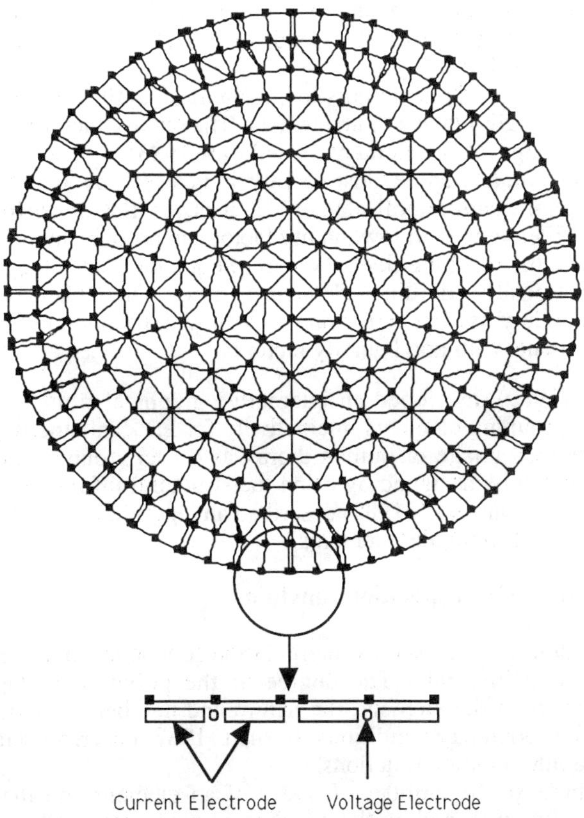

Figure 10.4 A two-dimensional circular finite-element model with 389 nodes, 536 elements, and 376 independent elements for a 32-electrode EIT system. 32 pairs of annular current and voltage electrodes cover 90% of the surface.

Interactive graphical mesh generator (IGMG)

When we design a finite element mesh for impedance imaging, we can use any *a priori* information about the internal structure of an object. Therefore, there is a need for an interactive graphical mesh generation tool for adding, removing, and grouping elements and also for easy change of boundary shape of an object. It could provide several interactive graphical tools which make it easy to design and modify a mesh. This mesh generator could be the front end of the EIT software package.

Automatic mesh generation and quality factor of element

Given the boundary definition of an object, the automatic mesh generator will generate a mesh in some predefined way, and the generated mesh can be modified later using the tools described above. Sabonnadiere and Coulomb (1987) describe several mesh generation techniques including meshing by block, grid superposition, frontal propagation, layer stacking and global decomposition. Heighway and Biddlecombe (1982) describe the two-dimensional automatic mesh generator used in the finite element electromagnetics package PE2D. Cendes *et al* (1983) describe the Delaunay triangulation algorithm.

Some automatic mesh generators include a mesh optimization method which is based on the quality factor of an element. The quality factor is determined by the size and shape of an element (Lindholm 1983). For a two-dimensional triangular element, any angle close to 180° indicates a low quality factor. For a two-dimensional quadrilateral element, if it is too flat or narrow, its quality factor is low. Elements with low quality factor can produce numerical problems when we solve the resulting linear system of equations since they may result in indefinite (not positive definite) element matrices. The Delaunay triangulation algorithm is widely used in generating a mesh with triangular elements since it generates elements with good quality factors.

Woo *et al* (1989) developed an interactive graphical finite mesh generator and tools for grouping elements interactively for EIT. This mesh generator can use a digitized CT image of human thorax as a background. Therefore, more realistic mesh can be designed by using the structural information contained in the CT image. Hussain *et al* (1989) described an algorithm to generate a uniform mesh composed of triangular elements.

10.3.2 Selection of interpolation functions

Usually polynomials are used as interpolation functions since they are easy to differentiate and integrate. The degree of the polynomial depends on the number of nodes in the element, the nature and number of unknowns at each node, and other boundary conditions. Burnett (1987) describes various kinds of elements and interpolation functions.

We can increase the number of nodes of an element and the order of the interpolation function and/or the number of elements until we achieve the required accuracy. For example, we can use a six-node triangular element with a quadratic interpolation function or we can divide the triangular element further into four small three-node triangular elements as shown in figure 10.5. In EIT, it is better to increase the number of elements rather than to increase the number of nodes of one element since the larger number of elements gives better spatial resolution of resistivity with the same number of total nodes (for the same amount of computation). We usually use a simple linear interpolation function for a triangular or isoparametric quadrilateral element.

10.3.3 Characterization of elements

Next, we evaluate the element matrix $\mathbf{y}$ which formulates solutions for individual elements. Huebner and Thornton (1975) describe four different

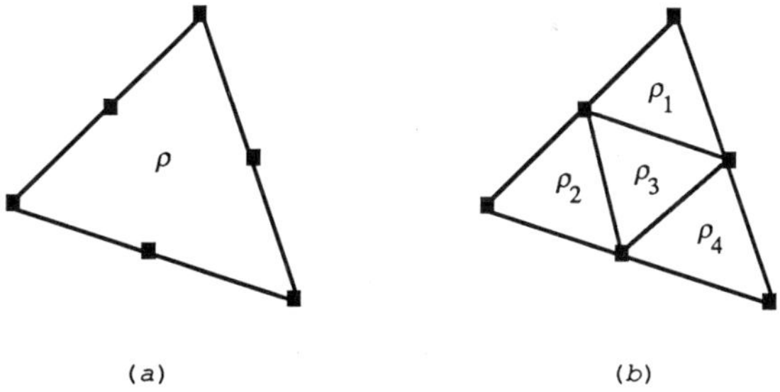

Figure 10.5 (*a*) A 6-node triangular element with a quadratic interpolation function, $V(x, y) = \alpha_1 + \alpha_2 x + \alpha_3 y + \alpha_4 x^2 + \alpha_5 y^2 + \alpha_6 xy$. (*b*) 4 small 3-node triangular elements with linear interpolation functions, $V(x, y) = \alpha_1 + \alpha_2 x + \alpha_3 y$. (*b*) gives better spatial resolution of resistivity than (*a*) for the same amount of computation time within the limit in the total number of elements described above.

methods for evaluating the element matrix. We use the variational approach where we use the constraint that the solution must have the minimal potential energy within each element with the given boundary conditions. Burnett (1987) describes more general methods called the methods of weighted residuals.

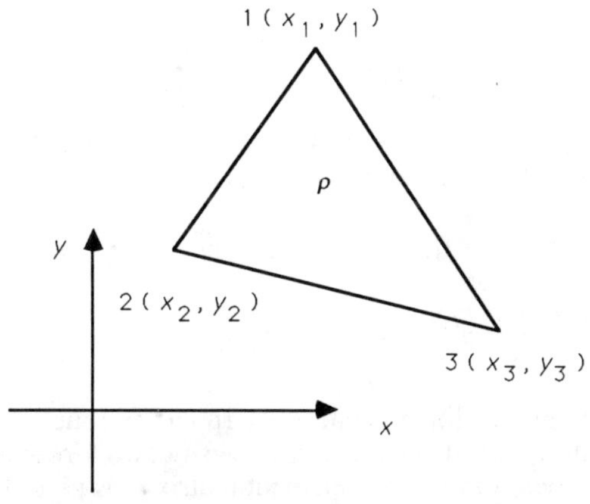

Figure 10.6 A typical triangular element, whose nodes i = 1, 2, 3 are located at coordinates x_i and y_i.

As an example, figure 10.6 shows a triangular element with resistivity ρ (Tong and Rossettos 1977). We choose a simple linear interpolation function as follows.

$$V(x, y) = \alpha_1 + \alpha_2 x + \alpha_3 y \tag{10.6}$$

where $V(x, y)$ is the voltage at (x, y) in the element, α_1 is the amount of voltage which doesn't change with position in the element, and $\alpha_2 x + \alpha_3 y$ is the amount of voltage which changes depending on the position in the element. This can be considered as the truncated Taylor series expansion of $V(x, y)$ in the element.

At each node,

$$V_1 = V(x_1, y_1) = \alpha_1 + \alpha_2 x_1 + \alpha_3 y_1$$

$$V_2 = V(x_2, y_2) = \alpha_1 + \alpha_2 x_2 + \alpha_3 y_2$$

$$V_3 = V(x_3, y_3) = \alpha_1 + \alpha_2 x_3 + \alpha_3 y_3 \qquad (10.7)$$

where 1, 2 and 3 are local node numbers of the element.

Then, we can determine α_1, α_2 and α_3 as follows:

$$\alpha_1 = \frac{a_1 V_1 + a_2 V_2 + a_3 V_3}{2\Delta}$$

$$\alpha_2 = \frac{b_1 V_1 + b_2 V_2 + b_3 V_3}{2\Delta}$$

$$\alpha_3 = \frac{c_1 V_1 + c_2 V_2 + c_3 V_3}{2\Delta} \qquad (10.8)$$

where $\Delta = \frac{x_2 y_3 - x_3 y_2 + x_3 y_1 - x_1 y_3 + x_1 y_2 - x_2 y_1}{2}$ = the area of the triangle, $a_1 = x_2 y_3 - x_3 y_2$, $b_1 = y_2 - y_3$, $c_1 = x_3 - x_2$ with the other a's, b's and c's obtained by cyclic permutation of the subscripts 1, 2 and 3. Then,

$$V(x, y) = V_1 f_1(x, y) + V_2 f_2(x, y) + V_3 f_3(x, y) \qquad (10.9)$$

where $f_i(x, y) = \frac{a_i + b_i x + c_i y}{2\Delta}$ $(i = 1, 2$ and $3)$.

The function, $f_i(x, y)$ is a dimensionless interpolation function and it has the value 1 at the ith node and 0 at the other two nodes. From the variational method, the (i, j) element of the 3×3 element matrix y_{ij} is given by

$$y_{ij} = \frac{1}{\rho} \iint_A \left(\frac{\partial f_i}{\partial x} \frac{\partial f_j}{\partial x} + \frac{\partial f_i}{\partial y} \frac{\partial f_j}{\partial y} \right) dA \qquad (10.10)$$

where A and dA denote the surface integral.

Then, the element matrix for the triangular element is

$$\mathbf{y} = \frac{1}{\rho 4\Delta} \begin{bmatrix} b_1^2 + c_1^2 & b_2 b_1 + c_2 c_1 & b_3 b_1 + c_3 c_1 \\ b_2 b_1 + c_2 c_1 & b_2^2 + c_2^2 & b_3 b_2 + c_3 c_2 \\ b_3 b_1 + c_3 c_1 & b_3 b_2 + c_3 c_2 & b_3^2 + c_3^2 \end{bmatrix}. \qquad (10.11)$$

Element matrices for other types of elements can be evaluated in the similar way. For quadrilateral and three-dimensional elements, we may need coordinate transformation and two-dimensional or three-dimensional numerical integration. Element matrices for various kinds of two-dimensional and three-dimensional elements are derived in the literature (Huebner and Thornton 1975, Tong and Rossettos 1977, Kim 1982, Burnett 1987).

10.3.4 Global node numbering and assembly of master matrix $\mathbf{Y}$

All nodes are numbered globally in the mesh. Also each node of an element has a local node number. Global node numbering could be done in an arbitrary way. However, the way we globally number the nodes greatly affects the amount of computation when we use the sparse matrix methods described in Chapter 11.

After we calculate element matrix $\mathbf{y}$ for each element, we assemble the master matrix $\mathbf{Y}$ to obtain the solution over the entire region. The basis of the assembly procedure is that the values of the field variable are the same at the nodes where elements are interconnected.

(1) Set $\mathbf{Y}_0 = \mathbf{0}$
(2) For i = first element to last element

$$\mathbf{Y}_i(m, n) = \mathbf{Y}_{i-1}(m, n) + \mathbf{y}(r, s)$$
$$m = \max(g_r, g_s),\ n = \min(g_r, g_s) \qquad (10.12)$$

where r and s are local node numbers of the ith element and g_r and g_s are global node numbers corresponding to r and s, respectively. Since the matrix $\mathbf{Y}$ is symmetric, this procedure generates only the lower triangular portion including the diagonal.

Now we have a linear system of equations, $\mathbf{Y}\boldsymbol{v} = \boldsymbol{c}$ where $\mathbf{Y}$ is the master matrix, $\boldsymbol{v}$ is the node voltage vector, and $\boldsymbol{c}$ is the node current vector. The master matrix , $\mathbf{Y}$ is $N \times N$ where N is the number of nodes in the finite element mesh.

10.3.5 Application of appropriate constraints

Since the rank of the master matrix is $N - 1$, we cannot directly solve the linear system of equations. Therefore, we need to set one reference node and modify the master matrix accordingly to have a rank of N. Furthermore, we should modify the master matrix and the current vector to impose the following two boundary conditions when they are available.

Reference node
We set one node as the reference node and set the voltage at the reference node to 0. This is done by setting the corresponding row and column of the master matrix to 0 with 1 at the diagonal and setting the corresponding element of the current vector to 0.

Dirichlet boundary condition (known surface voltages)
When we know some voltage values at the surface, we force the solution of the corresponding node voltages to have those known boundary values.

Neumann boundary condition (known surface currents)
When we know some current values at the surface (usually the injection currents), we set the corresponding elements of the current vector to those known values.

Now we have a uniquely solvable linear system equation with all boundary data in it.

$$\mathbf{Y}^* v = c^* \tag{10.13}$$

where $\mathbf{Y}^*$ is the modified master matrix and c^* is the modified current vector satisfying all constraints.

10.3.6 Solution of the matrix equation

Usually the master matrix is symmetric, positive definite, and very sparse. We can choose an efficient numerical technique based on the characteristics of the master matrix. The structure of the master matrix is determined by the global node numbering method. Therefore, careful node numbering is important for efficient solution of the resulting linear system equation.

Direct method
We can use Gaussian elimination or some variations of it. For the positive definite master matrix, Cholesky factorization with forward and back substitution might be the best direct method since it is numerically stable. In addition, the factorization methods are used in most of the sparse matrix algorithms.

By Cholesky factorization, we can express the master matrix as a product of a lower and an upper triangular matrix, $\mathbf{L}$ and $\mathbf{U}$. Since the master matrix is symmetric, $\mathbf{U}$ is the transpose of $\mathbf{L}$ ($\mathbf{U} = \mathbf{L}^T$). Then, the linear system of equations becomes $\mathbf{Y}^* v = \mathbf{L}\mathbf{L}^T v = c^*$. If we set $\mathbf{L}^T v = q$, we can first solve the equation $\mathbf{L}q = c^*$ for the vector q using forward substitution. Now, the voltage vector v can be obtained by solving the equation $\mathbf{L}^T v = q$ using back substitution. When we need to solve the linear system equation repeatedly for the same master matrix with different current vectors, this method is fast since we don't have to factorize the master matrix again (Tong and Rossettos 1977).

Iterative method
We can also use some iterative methods such as Gauss–Seidel or Successive Overrelaxation (SOR). These methods are faster than direct methods for certain types of matrices. We can use minimization techniques such as the conjugate gradient method to solve the linear system equation. This method is good when the size of the master matrix is very large. Depending on the characteristics of the master matrix, iterative methods can be faster than direct methods if we do not use any sparse matrix algorithm.

Since the required computation time for the solution of the linear system equation is very large, efficient numerical technique is essential.

10.3.7 Sparse matrix algorithm

Since the master matrix is very sparse, we can reduce the computation time significantly by using a sparse matrix algorithm together with a good node renumbering scheme. Most of the sparse matrix algorithms are based on the factorization method and they usually use row- or column-linked lists instead of simple two-dimensional arrays for the storage and manipulation of the matrix. Efficient sparse matrix algorithms do not compute any trivial computations such as multiplication by 0 and minimize the number of nontrivial computations. Chapter 11 discusses sparse matrix techniques and other computational topics related with reconstruction algorithms.

10.3.8 Examples

Figure 10.7 shows the injection current and the calculated voltages on the periphery of a two-dimensional circular computer model with 17 nodes, 20 triangular elements and 12 electrodes. Depending on the resistivity distributions of the model, the voltages on the periphery are different for the same injection current, $I(\theta) = \cos\theta$, where $0 < \theta < 2\pi$ is the angle around the circle. Note that the calculated voltage is highest at $\theta = 135^\circ$, over the high-resistivity object in figure 10.7(*e*) and (*f*).

Figure 10.8 shows the node voltages and current density vectors in each element for the same injection current as in figure 10.7. This model has 53 nodes, 80 triangular elements, and 24 electrodes. If this model were homogeneous with a resistivity of 100 Ω cm, then the spatial cosine distribution of injection current should have produced a uniform current density. Figure 10.8 shows the distortion of the current density due to the 370 Ω cm object at the center.

10.4 BACKPROJECTION BETWEEN EQUIPOTENTIAL LINES

10.4.1 Basic backprojection

This method is called backprojection between equipotential lines since they backproject the potential difference between two equipotential lines on the surface to the resistivity value in the inside area between those two equipotential lines (Barber *et al* 1983).

$$\rho = \rho_0 \frac{(V_i - V_j)_{\text{measured}}}{(V_i - V_j)_{\text{expected}}}. \tag{10.14}$$

As mentioned in Section 1.3 and figure 1.4, they average ρ over the entire image after all projection angles. This averaged image is then filtered by a ramp filter to reduce the blurring inherent in backprojection. They use the neighboring method for the data collection. Figure 8.1 shows the neighboring method and the equipotential lines in a homogeneous medium.

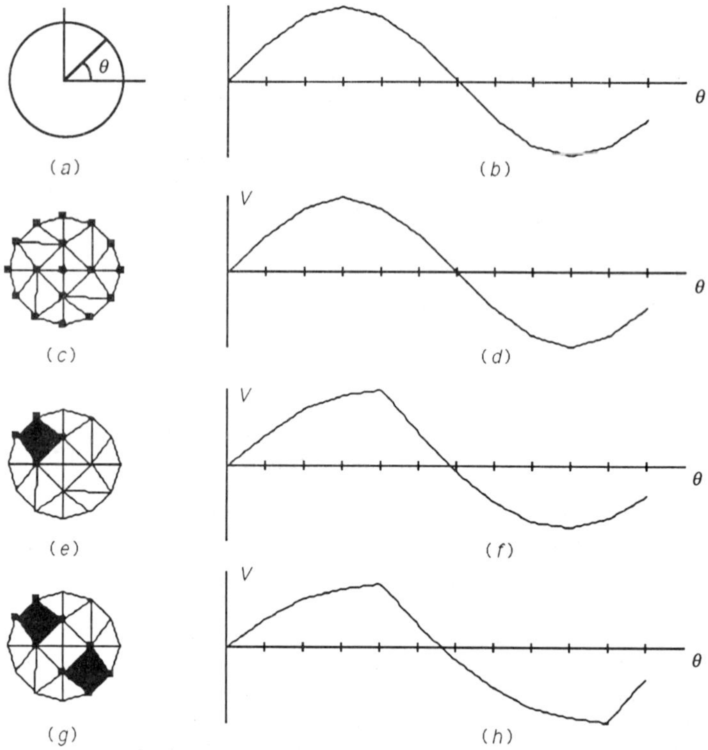

Figure 10.7 Calculated surface voltages for 3 different resistivity distributions with the same injection current, $I(\theta) = \cos\theta$. Background is 100 Ω cm and objects (black) are 370 Ω cm.

10.4.2 Fast filtered backprojection method

Under the assumption that the unknown resistivity distribution is close to a known reference resistivity distribution, there is an approximately linear relationship between the perturbation of the measured surface voltage gradients from those of the reference distribution and the logarithm of the resistivity perturbation from the reference distribution.

Barber and Brown (1986) and Barber and Seagar (1987) developed a fast filtered backprojection method for the reconstruction of the logarithm of the resistivity and Eyuboglu (1988) described the method in detail. They also argued that the neighboring method is best for their reconstruction method.

Computation of equipotential lines

For the circular, homogeneous, isotropic medium, the equipotential lines can be calculated by analytically solving Laplace's equation for given boundary conditions. However, Barber and Brown (1986) used a different approximate

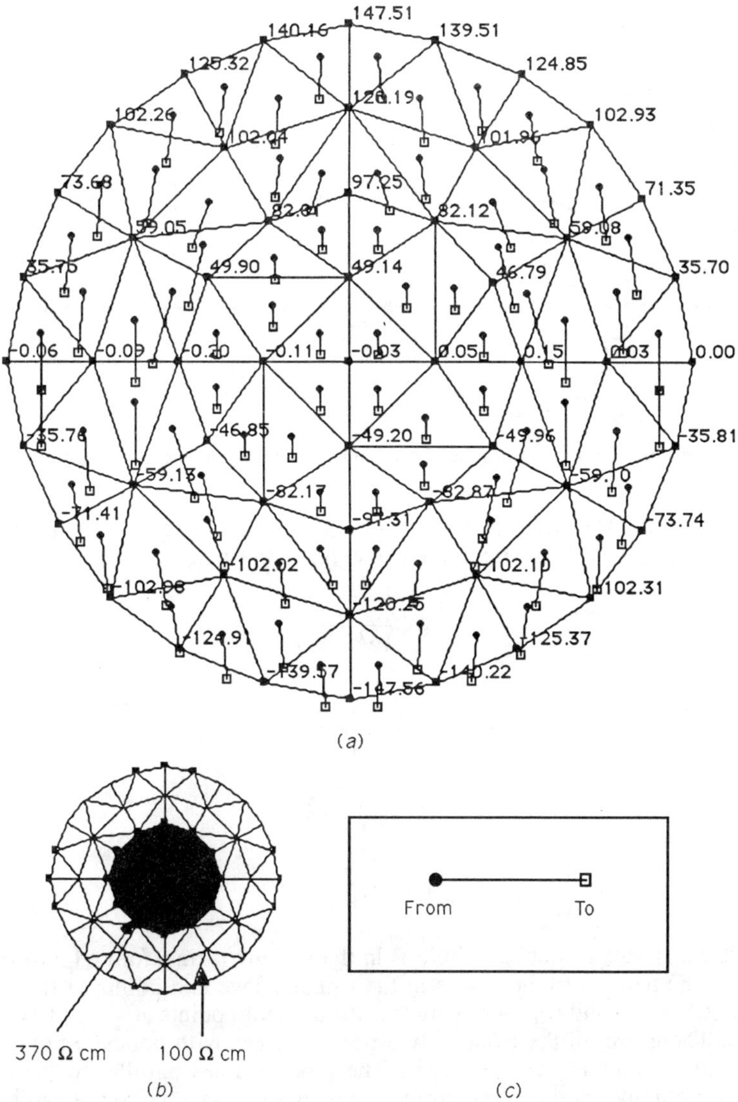

Figure 10.8 Calculated node voltages and electric current densities of elements for the same injection current as figure 10.7.

method of finding the equipotential lines in developing the backprojection reconstruction algorithm.

Assuming that the distance between two adjacent driving electrodes (2τ) is very small, they considered the drive pair of electrodes as a current dipole.

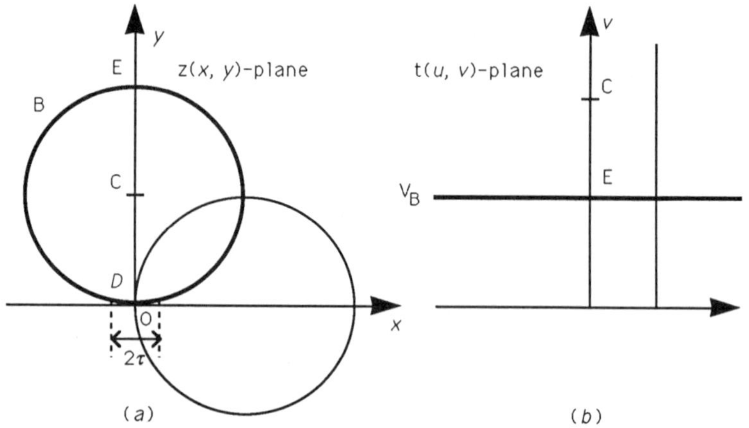

Figure 10.9 Conformal transformation between a circular region and a semi-infinite region.

Then, under the following conformal transformation, the z(x, y) plane in figure 10.9(a) can be transformed into the t(u, v) plane in figure 10.9(b).

$$x = \frac{u}{(u^2 + v^2)}$$

$$y = \frac{v}{(u^2 + v^2)}$$

$$u = \frac{x}{(x^2 + y^2)}$$

$$v = \frac{y}{(x^2 + y^2)} \cdot \qquad (10.15)$$

Under this transformation, circle B in the z-plane is transformed into straight line (v = E) parallel to the u-axis in the t-plane. Two end points of the current dipole ((0, 0 – τ) and (0, 0 + τ)) are transformed into points at $-\infty$ and $+\infty$ of the u-axis. Therefore, in the t-plane, two point charges with opposite polarity are placed at $-\infty$ and $+\infty$ of the u-axis. The straight lines parallel to the u-axis become field lines and are transformed into circles tangential to the x-axis at the point O in the z-plane. Similarly, equipotential lines which are perpendicular to the u-axis in the t-plane are transformed into the circular lines passing through the point O in the z-plane. If the dipole strength is m, then the equipotential lines are the lines passing through points at which

$$V = \frac{mx}{(x^2 + y^2)} \qquad (10.16)$$

is constant. This method is called the dipole approach and results in significant error close to the electrodes when the gap between the drive electrodes (2τ) is not sufficiently small.

Backprojection along equipotential lines

In figure 10.10(a), let $V_u(\Phi)$ be the potential measured at a point Q(Φ) on the boundary B from a homogeneous resistivity (ρ_u) medium S. Let $V_m(\Phi) = V_u(\Phi) + \Delta V(\Phi)$ be the potential measured at the same point after the resistivity of the medium has changed from ρ_u to $\rho_u + \Delta\rho_u$. Since the change in the boundary voltage is related to the change in the resistivity of the medium,

$$\frac{V_m(\Phi)}{V_u(\Phi)} \approx \frac{\rho_u + \Delta\rho}{\rho_u}. \tag{10.17}$$

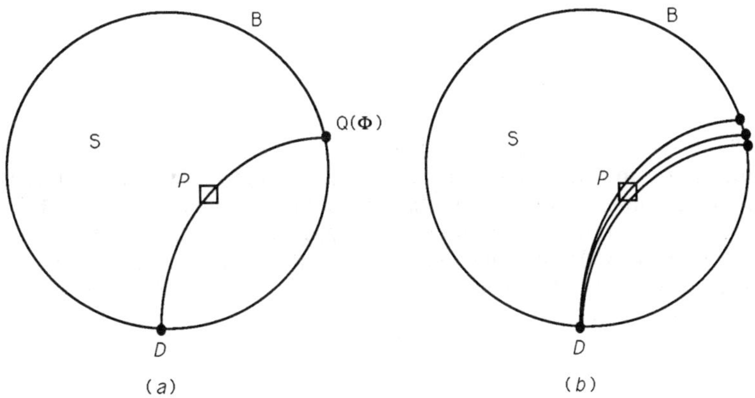

Figure 10.10 Backprojection of boundary voltage measurements.

Taking the natural logarithm of both sides and assuming that $\Delta V(\Phi) \ll V_u(\Phi)$, $\Delta\rho_u \ll \rho_u$, and therefore the shape of the equipotential lines are not changed significantly, the above equation becomes

$$\frac{\Delta V(\Phi)}{V_u(\Phi)} \approx -\frac{\Delta\rho}{\rho_u}. \tag{10.18}$$

Hence, the normalized boundary voltage change is backprojected into the image value of the pixel P which lies on the equipotential line ending at the point Q(Φ). Let $\boldsymbol{g}(D)$ be a vector of the normalized boundary voltage change for drive pair D and p be the image value of the pixel P. Then,

$$p = \boldsymbol{w}(PD)\,\boldsymbol{g}(D) \tag{10.19}$$

where $\boldsymbol{w}(PD) = [0, 0, \dots, w_j, 0, \dots, 0]$ is the backprojection vector for the pixel P, the drive pair D, and the jth voltage measuring electrode pair. w_j is a weighting factor for angular uniformity described in the next section. Since equation (10.19) holds for all pixels, we have

$$p(D) = \mathbf{W}(D)\, g(D) \qquad (10.20)$$

where $\boldsymbol{p}(D)$ is a vector of image values of all pixels and $\mathbf{W}(D)$ is a matrix whose rows are $\boldsymbol{w}(PD)$.

In practice, a pair of current injection electrodes (D) is not actually a dipole since 2τ is not sufficiently small. Therefore, to be more realistic, they move the dipole by small angles and find new equipotential lines originating from the new dipoles and passing through the pixel P. Then, different boundary potentials at the ending points of the new equipotential lines are backprojected into the pixel. In addition, since more than one equipotential line passes through a pixel due to the finite size of the pixel (figure 10.10(b)), corresponding boundary potentials are also backprojected appropriately into the pixel.

Since they use 16 electrodes, there are 16 drive pairs. The final image $\boldsymbol{p}$ is obtained as follows:

$$p = \sum_{D=1}^{16} p(D) = \mathbf{W}\, g. \qquad (10.21)$$

Weighting factors for angular uniformity

Assuming that the electrodes are equally spaced, the equipotential lines are not circularly symmetric for all pixels except the one at the center. Hence the weights of each equipotential line for backprojection should be different for all pixels other than the middle one. Based on the conformal transformation between a central point and an offset point (Seagar *et al* 1987), the weight w_j is computed as follows:

$$w_j = \frac{l - d^2}{l^2} \qquad (10.22)$$

where l and d are shown in figure 10.11.

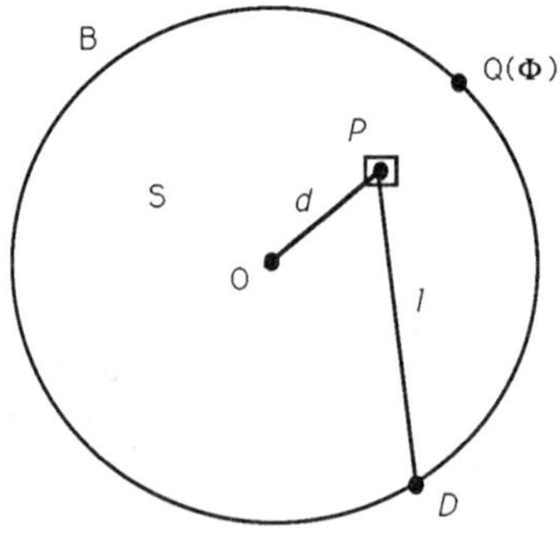

Figure 10.11 Computation of backprojection weight.

Filtering

Seagar *et al* (1987) show that the spatial resolution depends on the location of an object in the circular medium. In order to minimize the artifacts due to the severe position dependence of the spatial resolution of the reconstructed image, they developed a restoration filter empirically. They first applied a nonlinear radial transformation to the image to make the filtration problem position independent. They filtered the image with a position-independent resolution-restoring filter. Then, they applied the inverse radial transform to the result. The nonlinear radial transform and inverse transforms are

$$s = \tanh(r) \tag{10.23}$$

$$r = 0.5 \ln \frac{1+s}{1-s} \tag{10.24}$$

where r is the radial distance in the original image and s is the radial distance in the transformed image. The resolution-restoring filter they used was designed empirically and not described in detail.

Filtered backprojection

Let $\mathbf{E}$ denote the filtering operation and q be the final reconstructed image. Then,

$$q = \mathbf{E}\,p = \mathbf{E}\,\mathbf{W}\,g = \mathbf{T}^{-1}\,g. \tag{10.25}$$

Here, the backprojection and the filtering can be combined into a single filtered backprojection since the reconstruction algorithm is linear.

Figure 10.12 shows the reconstruction of a 1 cm cylindrical perspex object imaged in a shallow dish of saline using a 16-electrode system. Barber and Brown (1986) estimated that 5% of spatial resolution might be achievable by improving their reconstruction algorithm.

(*a*) (*b*)

Figure 10.12 Reconstruction of experimental data. The objects are at (*a*) the center of the field of view and (*b*) 5 cm from the center of the field of view. The dish (field of view) is 15 cm in diameter (Barber and Brown 1986).

10.4.3 Iterative equipotential lines method

The equipotential line method is a noniterative method. The image is presented after corrections have been made for all measurements. Yorkey *et al* (1987a) implemented the iterative equipotential line method. They also iteratively calculated the equipotential lines after each projection angle since the original equipotential lines are no longer valid after a single correction of the resistivity. They showed better performance of the iterative equipotential lines method over the noniterative one.

Ider *et al* (1987) implemented the iterative backprojection method. Starting from the homogeneous resistivity distribution, at the end of each iteration, they solved a forward problem using the updated resistivity values to compute new equipotential lines. They used the FEM to solve the forward problem. They developed a mesh with 1016 triangular elements and 541 nodes which can be adapted to a given boundary shape. Ider *et al* (1988) determined the position of electrodes using 16 ultrasonic transducers for their iterative equipotential method. Using a 16-electrode data acquisition system with a 12 bit ADC, they reconstructed a static resistivity image of an insulator in a circular phantom. They argued that their system is capable of reconstructing static images with conductivity contrast better than 20% and about 10% spatial resolution. They also argued that iteration is essential in producing static images by the backprojection between equipotential lines method.

10.4.4 Sensitivity coefficient method in backprojection

Breckon and Pidcock (1987) defined a sensitivity matrix and pointed out that the backprojection between equipotential lines method only uses the diagonal elements of the matrix. They suggested that the backprojection method might be improved by utilizing other sensitivity values since they are not negligible. Based on their suggestions, Kotre (1989) developed a backprojection algorithm which uses all sensitivity coefficients as weights.

From figure 10.13, assuming that $\delta\rho(x, y)$ is small, a sensitivity coefficient is defined as

$$S_{m,n,x,y} = \frac{\delta V(m, n)}{\delta\rho(x, y)} = \int_{e} \nabla\phi_m \cdot \nabla\phi_n \, dS \tag{10.26}$$

where e denotes the integration over the area of the element.

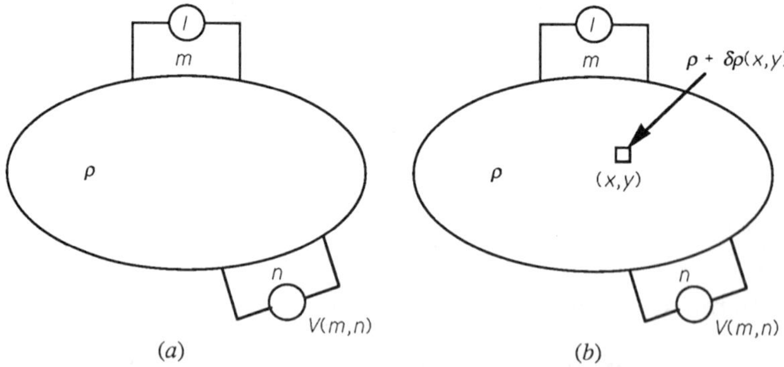

Figure 10.13 Schematic diagram showing the four-electrode method applied to the collection of impedance tomographic data in (*a*) a bounded volume of uniform resistivity, and (*b*) a bounded volume where one volume element has a changed resistivity (Kotre 1989).

The sensitivity matrix can be computed in the same way as the Jacobian matrix is computed in the modified Newton–Raphson method using the FEM (Section 10.7). Also, we can compute the sensitivity matrix from the analytic solution of Laplace's equation for the homogeneous resistivity distribution. Then, Kotre (1989) computed the pixel values $P(x,y)$ by

$$P(x, y) = \sum_{m=1}^{M} \sum_{n=1}^{N} S_{m,n,x,y} \ln\left[\frac{V'(m, n)}{V(m, n)}\right] \tag{10.27}$$

in his single-pass reconstruction algorithm.

Figure 10.14 shows reconstructed images of a Perspex/aluminium rod phantom and a human chest section. Proper use of the sensitivity matrix will improve the image quality of the backprojection method. However, this algorithm would produce less accurate images compared to an iterative nonlinear reconstruction algorithm though it has the advantages of speed and stability. Also, depending on the way that the sensitivity matrix is computed and used in the image reconstruction, different versions of similar algorithms are possible.

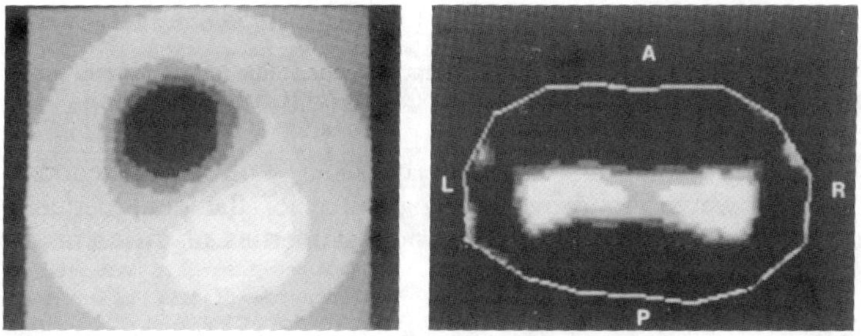

(*a*) (*b*)

Figure 10.14 Reconstructed images of (*a*) Perspex/aluminium rod phantom, and (*b*) human chest section. The image in (*b*) shows the changes in resistivity between expiration and inspiration. The light areas denote regions where a large change has occurred (Kotre 1989).

10.4.5 Dual-frequency imaging

Dielectric constant and electrical conductivity of human tissues change depending on the frequency. The conductivity of liver increases by 17% between 100 and 150 kHz. The conductivities of kidney and muscle also increase by 9 and 7%, respectively, between 100 and 150 kHz. Griffiths and Ahmed (1987) suggested an EIT system using two frequencies. They used the backprojection method in the computer simulation using 100 and 150 kHz for injection current. They used a measurement at one frequency as a reference to a measurement at another frequency to reconstruct a dual-frequency static image using the change in conductivity with frequency. They backprojected the difference between voltages at 100 and 150 kHz and showed that liver and kidney appeared most distinctly on the static dual frequency difference image due to their comparatively large dependency of conductivity on frequency.

Griffiths and Zhang (1989) used two frequencies, 40.96 and 81.92 kHz in their dual-frequency EIT system. From an *in-vitro* experiment using a cylindrical phantom with 16 stainless steel electrodes, they reconstructed a dual-frequency image of 200 g of porcine liver using the real part of the voltage measurement (resistivity image) as shown in figure 10.15. Because of systematic measurement errors (probably due to stray capacitance), they had to subtract the dual-frequency image of porcine liver from the dual-frequency image of the homogeneous saline phantom to cancel out the effect of error in the image. They also showed a dual-frequency image of the human abdomen *in-vivo* showing the erector spinae muscles for which conductivity increases by up to 50% between 40.96 and 81.92 kHz.

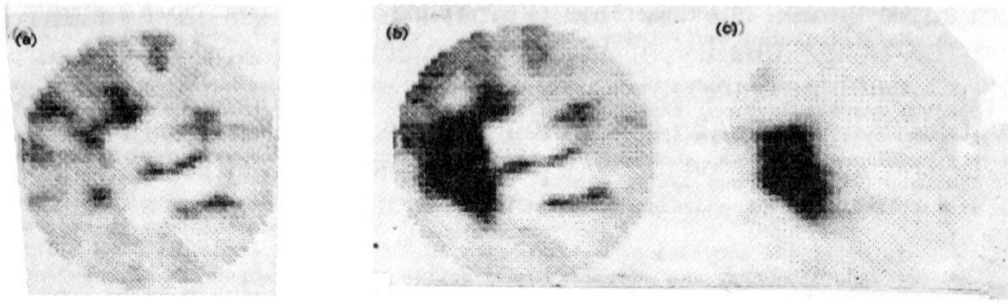

(*a*) (*b*) (*c*)

Figure 10.15 Dual-frequency image of (*a*) homogeneous saline and (*b*) saline with porcine liver immersed. (*c*) Difference between images (*a*) and (*b*) (Griffiths 1989).

Dual-frequency imaging can also be used with other reconstruction algorithms. However, to prove the feasibility of the dual-frequency EIT imaging, further research on the electrical properties of different tissues is required.

10.4.6 Discussion

The fast filtered backprojection method is based on the assumptions that the object has a circular boundary with equally spaced electrodes and is two-dimensional. Also, this method assumes that the resistivity distribution to be reconstructed is close to the reference resistivity distribution. In spite of those assumptions, this method rapidly produces useful difference images and is being used in various clinical applications. However, the main drawback of this method is that it can not reconstruct static images.

Barber and Brown (1988a) argued that this method is fairly immune to random electrode placement errors. Figure 10.16(*a*) shows a reconstructed image without electrode positioning error. Figure 10.16(*b*) shows an image of the same object with randomly placed electrodes for the measurement data set but not for the reference data set. Figure 10.16(*c*) shows an image of the same object with the same randomly displaced electrodes for both the measurement and the reference data set. The image in figure 10.16(*c*) is as good as the image in figure 10.16(*a*). However, sometimes it might be very difficult to keep the same electrode placement between the measurements of the two data sets. In such a case, the reconstructed image could be useless like the one in figure 10.16(*b*).

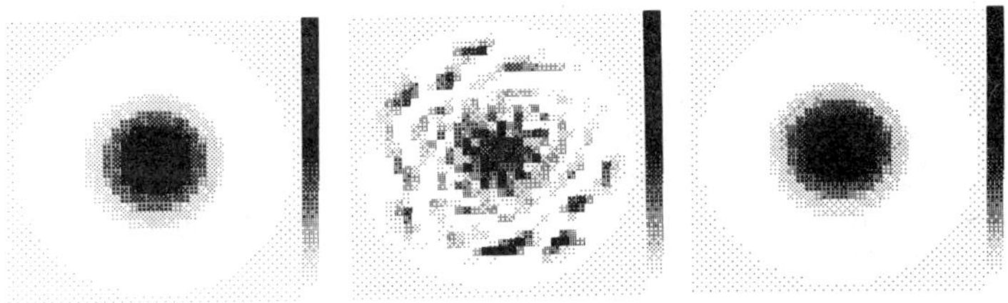

(*a*) (*b*) (*c*)

Figure 10.16 Effect of electrode position error on reconstructed image. (*a*) No error. (*b*) Random error in measurement data set but no error in reference data set. (*c*) Same random error in both measurement and reference data set (Barber and Brown 1988a).

The iterative backprojection method can provide more accurate images compared to the noniterative method at the expense of more computation time. Use of all sensitivity values in the sensitivity matrix is promising in improving the image quality of the backprojection method. Also, dual-frequency imaging might provide a kind of static image if problems in instrumentation are solved.

10.5 PERTURBATION METHOD

This method is based on the application of voltage and measurement of current. After Kim *et al* (1983) applied constant voltage on one large voltage electrode, they calculated the perturbation matrix by changing the resistivity of one element and calculated the change of currents at current-measuring electrodes using the FEM. They backprojected the percent change in currents caused by objects inside using the perturbation matrix.

Yorkey *et al* (1987b) developed an improved perturbation technique and recently Kim *et al* (1987) modified the perturbation method. However, they generally agree that the current-injection method is better than the voltage-application technique in obtaining a more accurate resistivity distribution.

10.5.1 Kim *et al*'s method

Formation of perturbation matrix

First, they calculated the exit currents for a particular projection angle with a homogeneous resistivity distribution. Then, they increased the resistivity of one element by a factor of ten, and calculated the change in exit currents in all the current-measuring electrodes for this projection angle. They repeated the same procedure for different projection angles. The normalized value of the amount of the change in exit current is the sensitivity value of the element with respect to the current-measuring electrode for the projection angle. Finally they calculated the perturbation matrix, $\mathbf{T}(E \times C \times P)$, where E is the number of elements, C is the number of current electrodes, and P is the number of projection angles.

Constraints
They stored only the integer portion of T_{ijl} to reduce the storage requirement and permitted corrections only within the central region by setting the sensitivity value of the outermost elements to zero. When the resistivities of the outermost elements were allowed to change with nonzero sensitivity values, the reconstruction diverged since the sensitivity values there are at least an order of magnitude larger than those at the center.

Backprojection after each projection angle
After measuring exit currents with an object inside for each projection angle, they backprojected the percent change in exit currents due to the object using the perturbation matrix as follows:

$$\rho_i{}^n = \rho_i{}^{n-1} + k \frac{\sum_{j=1}^{C} RC_{jl}{}^n \, T_{ijl} \;\, \rho_i{}^{n-1}}{\sum_{j=1}^{C} |T_{ijl}|} \tag{10.28}$$

where k is the overrelaxation factor, T_{ijl} is the sensitivity of the ith element in the jth current electrode at the lth projection angle, and $RC_{jl}{}^n$ is the percent difference between the predicted and actual exit current at the jth current electrode for the lth projection angle in the nth iteration.

10.5.2 Yorkey *et al*'s improved perturbation method

To improve the convergence behavior, Yorkey *et al* (1987b) corrected the resistivity values after they acquired all the data from all projection angles. This is similar to the simultaneous iterative reconstruction technique (SIRT) in the X-ray CT reconstruction technique whereas Kim *et al*'s method is similar to the algebraic reconstruction technique (ART) (Rosenfeld and Kak 1982).

$$\rho_i{}^n = \rho_i{}^{n-1} + k \frac{\sum_{i=1}^{P} \sum_{j=1}^{C} RC_{jl}{}^n \, T_{ijl} \;\, \rho_i{}^{n-1}}{\sum_{i=1}^{P} \sum_{j=1}^{C} |T_{ijl}|} . \tag{10.29}$$

They showed that the improved perturbation method is better for some resistivity distributions.

10.5.3 Kim *et al*'s modified method

Kim and Woo (1987) found that the sensitivity value is a function of element size, distance from the current-measuring electrode and background resistivity. The larger the element size, the closer to the current-measuring electrode, and the lower the background resistivity, the higher the sensitivity value. Based on this observation, they developed a modified perturbation method where they adjusted the resistivity during the backprojection based on a linearly decreasing function of distance from the current-measuring electrode. They also compared current measurements from other projections to properly determine the adjustment function. They defined columns of elements for each electrode pair and each projection as shown in figure 10.17. Backprojection along these columns is performed by updating the resistivity,

$$\rho_i{}^n = \rho_i{}^{n-1}k\left(\frac{C_{2\mathrm{pd}} - C_{1\mathrm{pd}}}{m-1}\,i + C_{1\mathrm{pd}}\right) + \rho_i{}^{n-1} \tag{10.30}$$

where m is the number of elements in the column, i is the element position in the column (between 0 and m), k is the overrelaxation factor, $\rho_i{}^n$ is the resistivity of the ith element in the nth iteration and $C_{1\mathrm{pd}}$, $C_{2\mathrm{pd}}$ are the percent differences between calculated and measured currents at electrodes C_1, C_2.

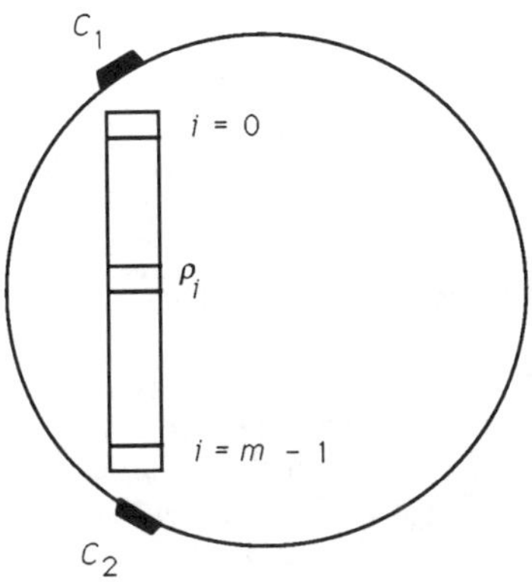

Figure 10.17 C_1 and C_2 are current-measuring electrodes, i is the position number, m is the number of elements in the column and ρ_i is the resistivity of element i.

10.5.4 Discussion

Figure 10.18 shows a three-dimensional representation of perturbation matrix entries. Since the perturbation matrix depends on the resistivity distribution, corrections based on the perturbation matrix calculated from the initial homogeneous resistivity distribution are no longer valid after corrections are made in the resistivity distribution. However, Yorkey *et al* (1987b) found no improvement when they calculated a new perturbation matrix after each iteration.

10.6 DOUBLE CONSTRAINT METHOD

Wexler *et al* (1985) developed a reconstruction method called the double constraint method. This method solves the Poisson's equation by the FEM using

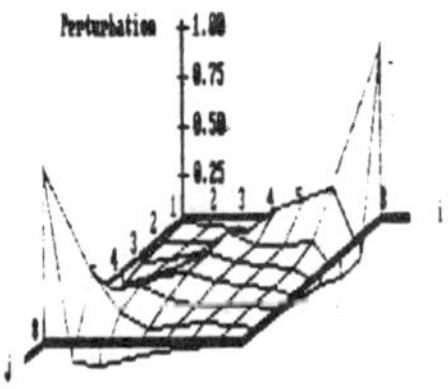

Figure 10.18 A three-dimensional representation of the perturbation matrix entries for the current exiting the lower-left-corner electrode of the computer model when the upper-right-corner electrode is connected to a voltage source and the remaining electrodes are grounded. The height represents the change in current normalized by the original current for a tenfold change in the resistivity of the element (i, j). A positive perturbation means an increase in resistivity in that element would cause the measured current to increase. Note how the edge elements cause much more perturbation than central elements (Yorkey *et al* 1987b).

Neumann boundary conditions and Dirichlet boundary conditions successively in each iteration. Initially assuming a homogeneous resistivity distribution, it updates the resistivity distribution in each iteration by using the compatibility between the two boundary conditions for a given resistivity distribution.

10.6.1 Wexler *et al*'s double constraint method

Step 1 Calculation of voltage, V and current density, J with Neumann boundary conditions (currents at surface—injection currents)
We can solve the Poisson equation for the voltage values inside the region due to the injection currents using the FEM. The FEM calculates the voltage at each node. Then we can calculate the electric field intensity,

$$\boldsymbol{E} = -\nabla V. \tag{10.31}$$

Now the electric current density $\boldsymbol{J}$ in each element is given by

$$\boldsymbol{J} = \sigma \boldsymbol{E} = -\sigma \nabla V = -\rho^{-1} \nabla V \tag{10.32}$$

where σ is the conductivity and ρ is the resistivity of the element. In Section 10.3.8, there is a numerical example of the calculation of the voltage and the electrical current density in a two-dimensional circular finite element model (see figure 10.8).

The resistivity distribution used in this step is different from the actual resistivity distribution until the error between the calculated surface voltages and the measured voltages satisfies the stopping criterion. Therefore, the calculated electric current density distribution becomes closer to the actual current density distribution in each iteration even though they do not become identical.

In this step, we calculate the error between the calculated surface voltages and the measured voltages and go to step 2 if the error is larger than a certain small value (stopping criterion). Otherwise, we stop the iterative procedure and go to step 5 for the image display.

Step 2 Calculation of voltage, V and $-\sigma\nabla V$ inside with both Neumann and Dirichlet boundary conditions (injection currents and measured voltage data at surface)

In step 2, we solve the Poisson equation again for the voltage values inside the region using the measured surface voltage values as the Dirichlet boundary condition while using the same Neumann boundary condition. This produces more accurate estimates of the voltage values inside the region because the measured surface voltages used as boundary data change the voltage values at each node in the correct direction.

Step 3 Calculation of resistivity

The solution of the Poisson equation using one boundary condition (Neumann or Dirichlet) is unique. After we solve the equation for the voltage values using one type of boundary data, we can calculate the other type of boundary data from the solution. Therefore, the boundary conditions should be compatible for a given resistivity distribution. However, two solutions from step 1 and step 2 are not identical since we do not know the actual resistivity distribution.

In step 3, we calculate the new resistivity distribution from the minimization of the squared error between the electric current density of step 1 and that of step 2. The following equation defines the squared residual sum, R,

$$R = \sum_i \iiint_{v_i} (J_i + \sigma_i \nabla V_2) \cdot (J_i + \sigma_i \nabla V_2)\, dv \qquad (10.33)$$

where v_i and dv denote the volume integral over the element i, $\boldsymbol{J}_i$ is the calculated electric current density in the element i from step 1 and $-\sigma_i \nabla V_2$ is the electric current density in the same element from step 2.

Assuming homogeneous resistivity within one element, we calculate the new resistivity from the minimization of the squared residual sum,

$$\frac{\partial R}{\partial \sigma_i} = \iiint_{v_i} (2J_i \cdot \nabla V_2 + 2\sigma_i \nabla V_2 \nabla V_2)\, dv = 0 \qquad (10.34)$$

and

$$\sigma_i = \frac{1}{\rho_i} = \frac{-\iiint_{v_i} J_i \cdot \nabla V_2 dv}{\iiint_{v_i} \nabla V_2 \cdot \nabla V_2 dv}. \qquad (10.35)$$

Step 4 Final image processing and presentation
In this step, we can apply edge detection or other image enhancement techniques to the reconstructed image. Also we may need some image processing for a three-dimensional presentation.

10.6.2 Kohn *et al*'s relaxation of a variational method

Kohn and Vogelius (1987) suggested a reconstruction algorithm similar to Wexler *et al*'s. They found the relaxation of Wexler *et al*'s variational method. They argued that the relaxed problem is more efficient for practical calculation since the minimization of the relaxed functional on a coarse mesh is roughly equivalent to the minimization of the original one on a much finer mesh. Numerical testing is underway.

10.6.3 Discussion

Figure 8.10 shows the three-dimensional model used by Wexler *et al* (1985). Figure 10.19 shows the real image and reconstructed image after 1700 iterations using this method. This method needs many iterations since the effect of the Dirichlet boundary condition on the voltage values in step 2 is small. Wexler (1988) claimed that this method is not subject to matrix ill-conditioning compared to the method where minimization is applied to the boundary voltage error (such as in the Newton–Raphson method). Based on the experiment with a three-dimensional phantom, he argued that this method works in principle. However, he also said that improvement is needed to enhance the image quality and some scheme is needed to reduce the number of iterations. He suggested more accurate modeling of fields near the electrodes for image enhancement.

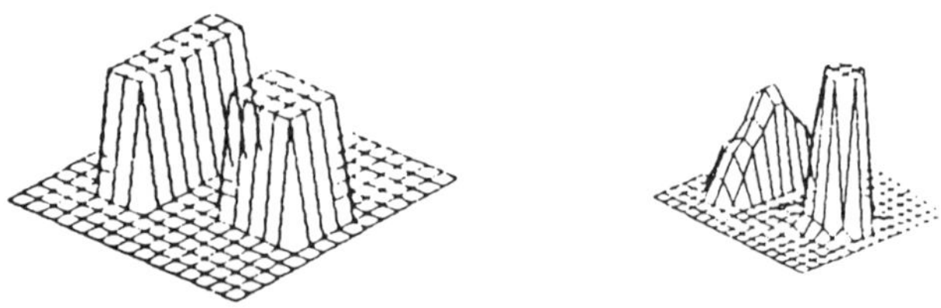

Figure 10.19 The actual image and the reconstructed image after 1700 iterations using the double constraint method (Wexler *et al* 1985).

10. 7 NEWTON–RAPHSON METHOD

The Newton–Raphson algorithm is an iterative reconstruction algorithm specifically developed for nonlinear problems. It is one of the most theoretically sound algorithms used in EIT. Yorkey *et al* (1986) described the algorithm in detail.

10.7.1 The measure of error

A direct measure of reconstruction error is to compare the real resistivity distribution with the reconstructed one. However, the real distribution is unknown. Thus, we can only take an indirect measure, that is, to compare the voltage responses of the resistivity distribution. If the voltage responses of the assumed resistivity distribution match those of the real distribution, we claim that the assumed distribution is the desired answer.

The error that we would like to minimize is called the objective function. There are many ways to define the function. Yorkey *et al* (1986) define it as the equally weighted mean square difference between the measured and estimated voltage responses,

$$\Phi(\rho) = (1/2)(f(\rho) - \boldsymbol{V}_0)^{\mathrm{T}}(f(\rho) - \boldsymbol{V}_0) \tag{10.36}$$

where $\boldsymbol{V}_0$ is the measured voltage, $f(\rho)$ the estimated voltage for a resistivity distribution ρ and T means transpose.

10.7.2 Newton–Raphson method

To find a ρ which minimizes Φ, we set its derivative to zero, i.e.,

$$\Phi'(\rho) = [f'(\rho)]^{\mathrm{T}}(f(\rho) - \boldsymbol{V}_0) = \boldsymbol{0} \tag{10.37}$$

where $[f'(\rho)]_{ij} = \partial f_i / \partial \rho_j$, and is called the Jacobian matrix.

We take the Taylor series expansion of $\Phi'(\rho)$ about an point ρ^k and keep the linear terms

$$\Phi'(\rho^{k+1}) \approx \Phi'(\rho^k) + \Phi''(\rho^k)\Delta\rho^k = \boldsymbol{0} \tag{10.38}$$

where

$$\rho^{k+1} = \rho^k + \Delta\rho^k. \tag{10.39}$$

The term Φ'' is called the Hessian matrix, expressed as

$$\Phi'' = [f']^{\mathrm{T}} f' + [f'']^{\mathrm{T}}\{\boldsymbol{I} \otimes [f - \boldsymbol{V}_0]\} \tag{10.40}$$

where $\otimes$ is the Kronecker matrix product. We omit the second term in the above equation, since f'' is difficult to calculate and relatively small. Therefore, we obtain

$$\Phi'' = [f']^{\mathrm{T}} f' \tag{10.41}$$

We substitute equations (10.41) and (10.37) into equation (10.38), and find the updating equation for ρ

$$\Delta\rho^k = -[f'(\rho^k)^{\mathrm{T}} f'(\rho^k)]^{-1}[f'(\rho^k)]^{\mathrm{T}}[f(\rho^k) - V_0]. \tag{10.42}$$

The above method is called either the modified Newton–Raphson method, or the Gauss–Newton method. Figure 10.20 shows the flow chart of the algorithm. We first guess a distribution, then calculate its theoretical voltage response for the given current distributions using the finite-element method. We subtract the calculated voltages from the measured voltages to obtain the objective function. If it is less than a criterion error, we take the guessed distribution as the desired distribution. If not, we update the distribution using equation (10.42). We repeat the above procedure until the stopping criterion is met.

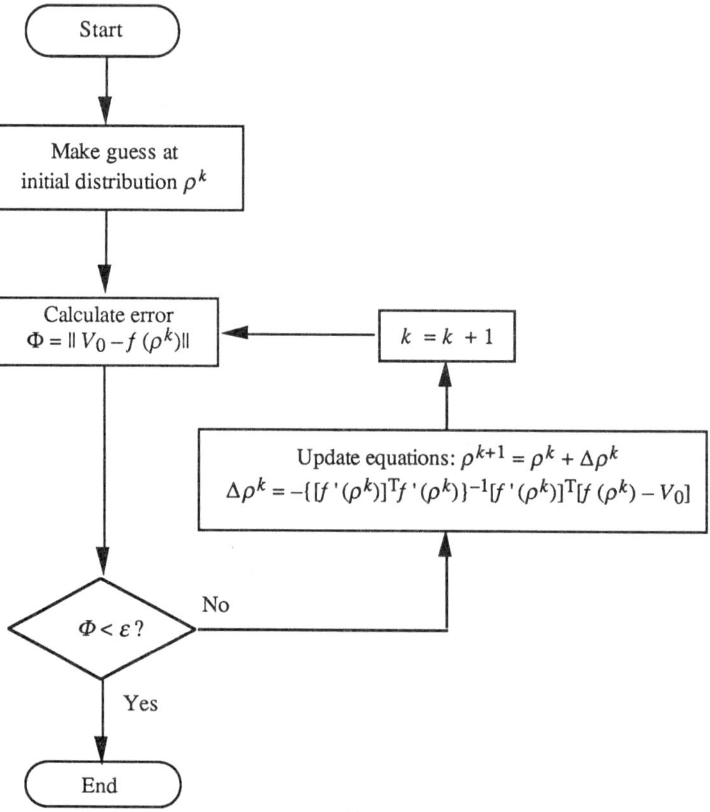

Figure 10.20 The Newton–Raphson algorithm performs k iterations to minimize the mean-squared error Φ.

Figure 10.21 shows the searching procedure of the Newton–Raphson algorithm in a scalar case. Since f is proportional to ρ, Φ is a quadratic function of ρ. We find its derivative Φ' which is a linear function. For the assumed distribution ρ^k, we evaluate the error Φ to determine if it is less than our criterion ε. If not, we find the slope of Φ', then update the assumed distribution along the direction opposite to the slope. In this linear case, we can find the solution in one step, as we know $\rho = \alpha(V/I)$, where α is a constant which measures the geometric shape of the medium.

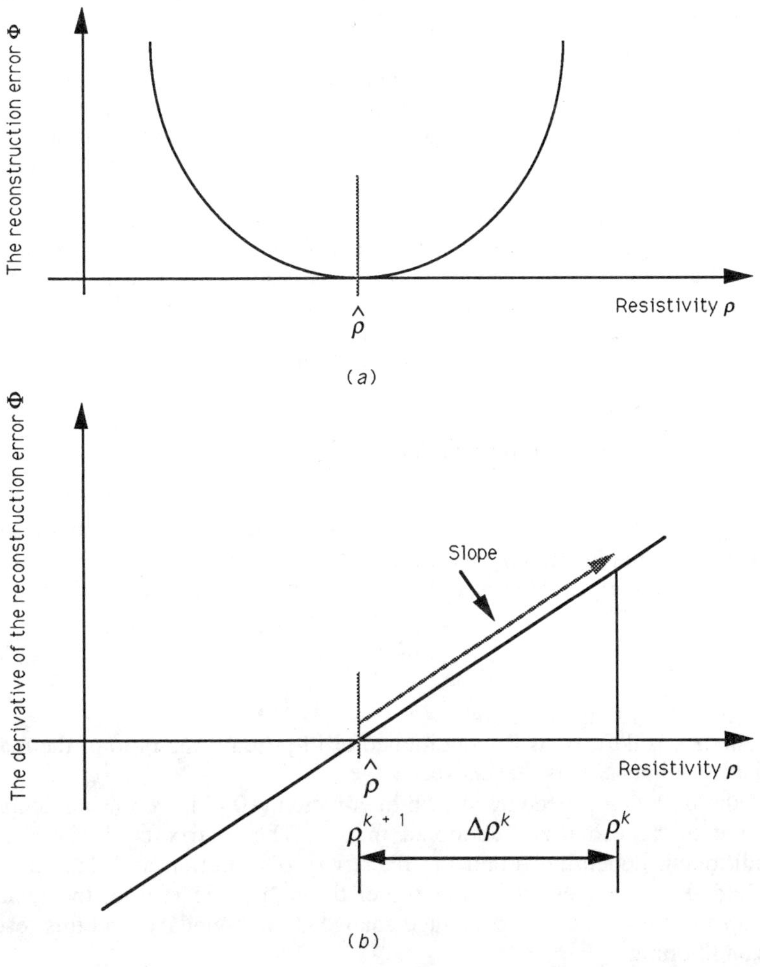

Figure 10.21 (*a*) The reconstructed error Φ is a quadratic function of ρ. (*b*) We find the slope of Φ', and update the resistivity value along the direction opposite to the slope.

The vector $f(\rho)$ denotes a collection of all voltage data, which should contain sufficient information about the resistivity distribution. The number of independent data measurements should be equal to or greater than the number of pixels of our image. This usually requires us to make several sets of measurements, with each set being the voltage response of one current distribution, which we call a projection.

The calculation of f and f' requires the use of the FEM, as described in Section 10.3. We first divide the media into many area elements, and assign each independent element an unknown representing the resistivity value of one pixel. We then establish a system function to describe the relationship among resistivity distribution, voltage and current. For each current distribution, we solve the system function to obtain its voltage response v_i, $i = 1$ to n, the number of projections. We simply stack the voltages from all the projections to form f, i.e., $f = [v_1^T\ v_2^T\ v_i^T \dots v_n^T]^T$.

The step size of the updating depends on the application, and is usually less than one to achieve guaranteed convergence. If the step size is too big, even though it may show fast convergence during the first few iterations, it would cause oscillation in the neighborhood of the solution. Equation (10.42) has a step size of unity.

The N–R algorithm's performance is well known for a quadratic function. In EIT, the voltages are nonlinear functions of the resistivity distributions instead of quadratic functions. Therefore the search may result in a local minimum, depending upon the initial guess of a resistivity distribution. We can avoid the problem by making an appropriate guess. In biomedical applications, we have sufficient prior knowledge to provide a good initial guess.

10.7.3 The ill-conditioning problem

The eigenvalues $\lambda(\mathbf{A}) = \{\lambda_1\lambda_2 \dots \lambda_n\}$ of an n by n matrix $\mathbf{A}$ are the n roots of its characteristic polynomial $p(z) = \det(z\mathbf{I} - \mathbf{A})$.

For the given eigenvalue λ_i, the nonzero vectors $\boldsymbol{x}$ that satisfy

$$\mathbf{A}\boldsymbol{x} = \lambda_i \boldsymbol{x} \tag{10.43}$$

are referred to as eigenvectors.

A matrix is defined as ill-conditioned or ill-posed if the ratio of the maximal and the minimal eigenvalues is very large.

In the updating procedure shown in equation (10.42), we must calculate the inverse of a normalized Jacobian matrix. The matrix could be very ill-conditioned, depending upon the resistivity distribution and data collection method. If the current does not travel through some region, the resistivity change does not yield much voltage change at the boundary, and this results in ill-conditioning.

Ill-conditioning causes the matrix inversion to be very inaccurate. It also causes the updating of equation (10.42) to be sensitive to measurement error. Both factors result in large reconstruction errors.

10.7.4 The adaptive method

Isaacson (1986) proposed a data collection method which achieves the maximal distinguishability δ. If we define the norm of the voltage difference $f(\rho^k) - V_0$

in equation (10.42) as signal, and the data collection errors described in Chapter 9 as noise, the method has the maximal signal-to-noise ratio (SNR) (Hua 1987). Therefore, this data set would result in a superior reconstructed image. Isaacson showed that the optimal current distributions are the eigenvectors of the largest eigenvalues of the impedance matrix **D**.

The matrix **D** in Section 8.6 has eigenvalues $\lambda_1, \lambda_2, \ldots, \lambda_n$ in a decreasing order, and eigenvectors $I_1, I_2, \ldots, I_n$, then the matrix can be decomposed into the following form:

$$\mathbf{D} = \lambda_1 I_1 I_1^{\mathrm{T}} + \lambda_2 I_2 I_2^{\mathrm{T}} + \ldots + \lambda_n I_n I_n^{\mathrm{T}}. \quad (10.44)$$

Using the iterative method in Section 8.6, we can find the dominant eigensystem λ_1 and I_1. We form another matrix **D**' as follows:

$$\mathbf{D}' = \mathbf{D} - \lambda_1 I_1 I_1^{\mathrm{T}} = \lambda_2 I_2 I_2^{\mathrm{T}} + \ldots + \lambda_n I_n I_n^{\mathrm{T}}. \quad (10.45)$$

Then using the algorithm again with **D**' substituted for **D**, we can obtain the dominant eigensystem of **D**', i.e., λ_2 and I_2. We repeat the above procedure to obtain the rest of the desired distributions.

The accumulated round-off error in the numerical implementation of the above procedure could result in inaccurate distributions. A small stopping error for the iterative process in Section 8.6 and accurate representation of the variables are necessary.

Figure 10.22 shows the block diagram of an adaptive system based on the optimal current method (Gisser *et al* 1987). We make an initial guess of the resistivity distribution. We then calculate the optimal currents which provide the best SNR. We measure the voltages from the real object impedance distribution, then use the Newton–Raphson algorithm to update the model resistivity distribution based on known currents and measured voltage data. Since the optimal current is resistivity-dependent, we need to recalculate the current distributions (Hua 1987) and repeat this procedure. We stop the iteration after the voltage error is small enough or the number of iterations exceeds a predefined value.

10.7.5 Static images from a phantom

Figures 10.23, 10.24 and 10.25 show reconstructed static images from a circular two-dimensional phantom using the modified Newton–Raphson method. These static images were reconstructed using the EIT system developed at the University of Wisconsin–Madison which uses 32 compound electrodes, 32 independent current sources, one voltmeter with 12 bit accuracy, the FEM and a Macintosh II as the host computer. Figure 10.23 shows the changes of images during image reconstruction using the modified Newton–Raphson method. Figure 10.24 shows three static images for three different objects. No postprocessing was done on these images though postprocessing could make images look better. Images in figure 10.25 were reconstructed using a different finite element mesh and regularization (Section 10.10).

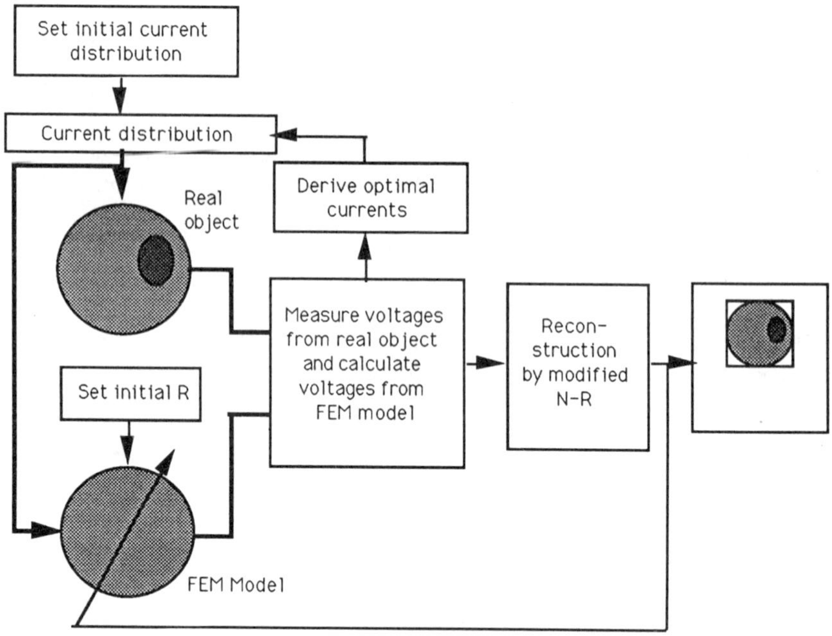

Figure 10.22 We use the FEM model to estimate the impedance distribution of the real object. We derive the optimal currents and apply them to both objects. We then measure the voltages from the real object and calculate the voltages from the FEM model. If the residual error is small enough, we stop. Otherwise, we update the estimated distribution by the modified Newton–Raphson method.

10.8 COMPENSATION THEOREM METHOD

10.8.1 Sensitivity theorem

Geselowitz's sensitivity theorem states how the voltage changes respond to resistivity changes. Figure 10.26 shows an impedance network. Apply a current source c_k to port k, resulting in the voltage V_i at port i. If the port j conductance y_i changes to $y_i + \Delta y_i$, the discrete version of sensitivity theorem (Murai and Kagawa 1985, Nakayama *et al* 1981) states that the voltage change at port i is

$$\Delta v_i = -c_k \Delta y_j \, z_{ij'} \, z_{kj} \qquad (10.46)$$

where z is the transfer impedance between the described ports, and j' denotes the changed port.

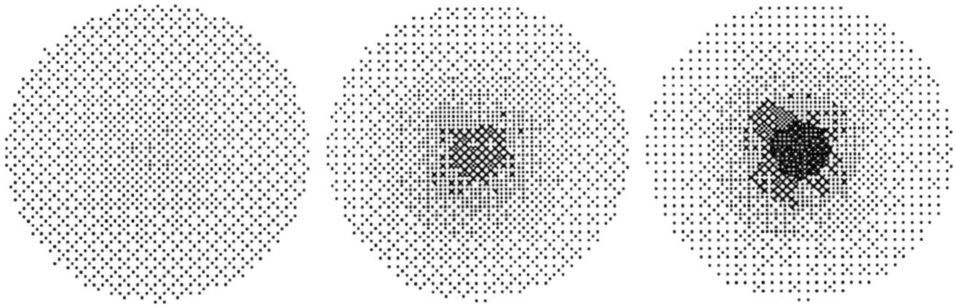

(*a*)

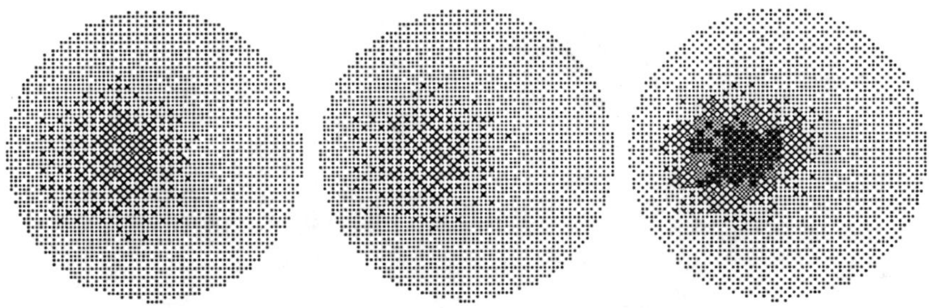

(*b*)

Figure 10.23 Images are improved as we use more iterations of the modified Newton–Raphson method. Images were obtained after 1, 2 and 20 iterations. (*a*) The object is an 8 cm diameter cylindrical insulator at the center of a 30 cm diameter two-dimensional circular phantom. (*b*) The object is an 8 cm diameter cylindrical insulator at an offset position inside the same phantom. Background is 100 Ω cm saline.

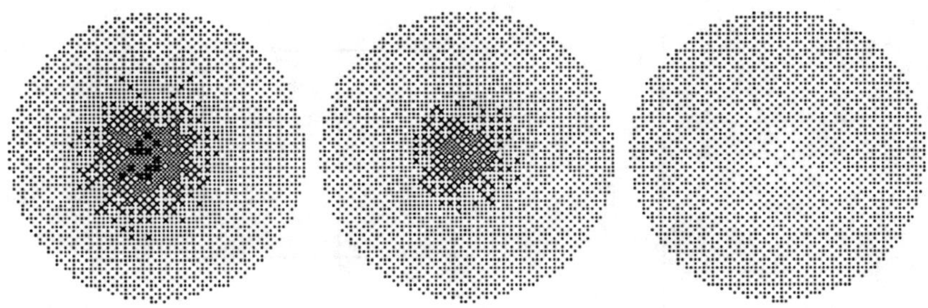

(*a*) (*b*) (*c*)

Figure 10.24 Reconstructed static images from a 30 cm diameter circular two-dimensional phantom using the modified Newton–Raphson method. The object is (*a*) an 8 cm diameter cylindrical insulator at the center, (*b*) a fist at the center, (*c*) a 5 cm cylindrical agar object at the center. Background is 100 Ω-cm saline.

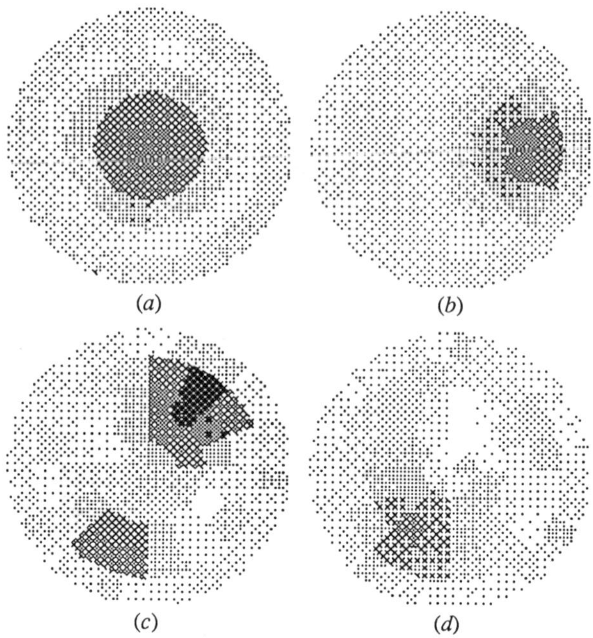

Figure 10.25 Reconstructed static images using different mesh and regularization. (a) An 8 cm diameter cylindrical insulator at the center, (b) An 8 cm diameter cylindrical insulator at an offset position, (c) two 8 cm diameter cylindrical insulators at offset positions, and (d) an 8 cm cylindrical insulator and a 5 cm cylindrical conductor at offset positions in the same phantom as figure 10.24. Background is 100 Ω cm saline.

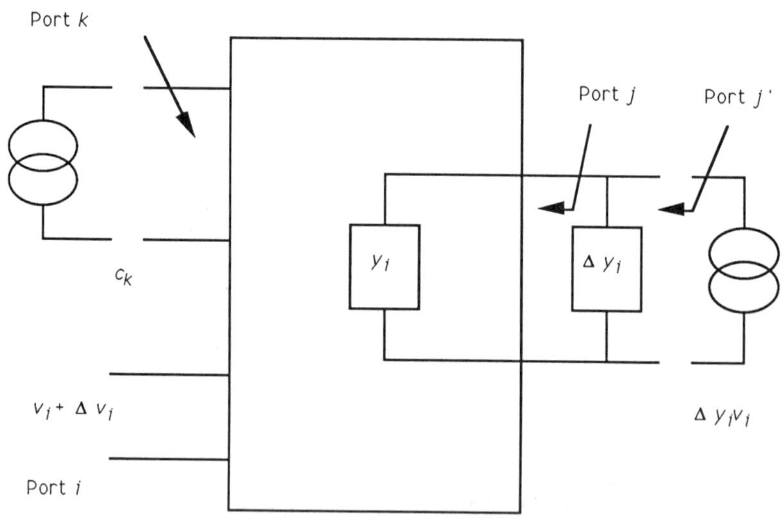

Figure 10.26 When we apply a current source to port k and an admittance $y_j + \Delta y_j$ the compensation theorem shows us how to calculate the resulting voltage at port j by removing the current source and applying a particular current source to port j'. We can use this theorem to calculate the Jacobian matrix more efficiently.

10.8.2 The compensation theorem algorithm

In the finite-element model, each element is made of L resistors with the resistivity value being $\rho_j s_l$, $l = 1$ to L, where ρ_j is the resistivity value and s_l is the FEM coefficient. A change in conductivity of an element causes changes of L resistor values, therefore, the corresponding voltage change at port i is the summation of the changes due to individual resistivity, as shown in the following equation:

$$\Delta v_i = -c_k \sum_{l=1}^{L} \Delta y_j(l) z_{ij'}(l) z_{kj}(l). \quad (10.47)$$

By replacing Δy_j with resistivity value ρ_j and FEM coefficient s_l, equation (10.47) becomes

$$\Delta v_i = -\Delta\sigma_j c_k \sum_{l=1}^{L} s_l z_{ij'}(l) z_{kj}(l). \quad (10.48)$$

When $\Delta\sigma_j$ approaches zero, $z_{ij'} = z_{ij}$. Substitute $\rho_j = \sigma_j^{-1}$, to obtain

$$\frac{\partial v_i}{\partial \rho_j} = \frac{1}{c_k \rho_j^2} \sum_{l=1}^{L} s_l v_{ij}(l) v_{kj}(l). \quad (10.49)$$

If there are M current sources at M ports, then equation (10.49) becomes

$$\frac{\partial v_i}{\partial \rho_j} = \sum_{k=1}^{K} \frac{1}{c_k \rho_j^2} \sum_{l=1}^{L} s_l v_{ij}(l) v_{kj}(l). \quad (10.50)$$

This forms the entry of the Jacobian matrix in equation (10.42). Therefore, the method essentially is the Newton–Raphson method which uses the compensation theorem to calculate the Jacobian matrix.

10.9 COMPARISON OF RECONSTRUCTION METHODS

Yorkey *et al* (1987a) used computer simulations to compare the performance of the different nonadaptive algorithms. Figure 10.27 shows the convergence of different methods for a given resistivity distribution. The Newton–Raphson and Compensation theorem algorithms converge to zero after four iterations. All the other methods have a residual error after 20 iterations, with the equipotential method performing the poorest.

Figure 10.28 shows the time for one iteration of each method. The standard Newton–Raphson method takes a long time for each iteration, approximately four times that of the compensation theorem method, while both methods require the same number of iterations.

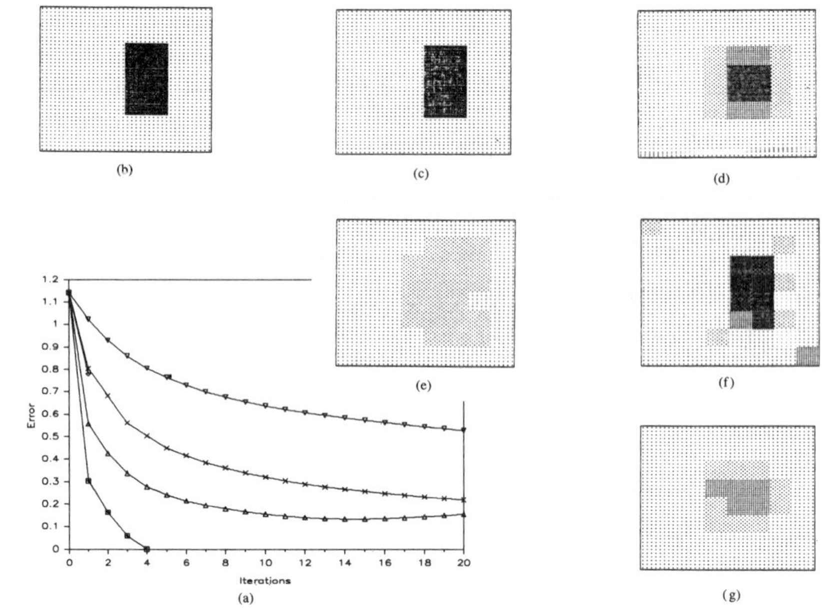

Figure 10.27 (*a*) The error in each iteration for the methods we outlined here. □ the standard method and, + compensation theorem method for calculating the Jacobian matrix. × perturbation method, ◊ equipotential, Δ iterative equipotential and ∇ double constraint. The equipotential method has a point only at the first iteration mark. Note both methods in computing the Jacobian matrix have the same errors, and the iterative equipotential method started to diverge. The final images for (*b*) standard and (*c*) compensation theorem method for calculating the Jacobian matrix. (*d*) Perturbation, (*e*) equipotential, (*f*) iterative equipotential, and (*g*) double constraint methods (Yorkey *et al* 1987a).

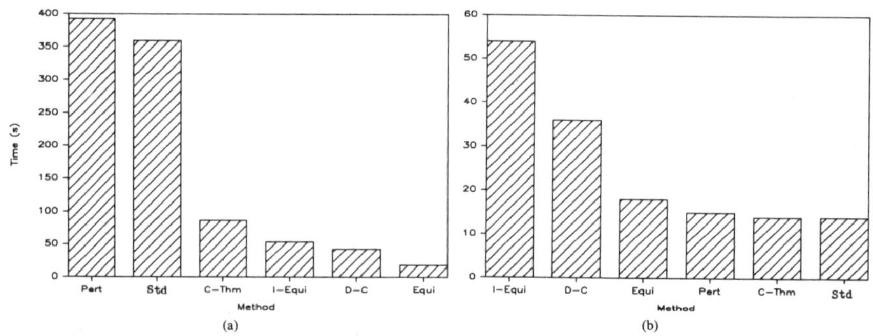

Figure 10. 28 (a) The time for one iteration of each method. For the equipotential method, this is the total time. Std: standard and C-Thm: compensation theorem method for calculating the Jacobian matrix. Pert: perturbation, Equi: equipotential, I-Equi: iterative equipotential, and D-C: double constraint method. (*b*) The time for one iteration of each method if we make all recomputations possible. Note now all methods take approximately the same time (Yorkey *et al* 1987a).

10.10 REGULARIZATION METHOD

The ill-conditioning degrades the performance of the Newton–Raphson algorithm for data contaminated with measurement error. The matrix $[f']^{T}[f']$ is a complicated function of current, voltage and the unknown resistivity distribution. Therefore, improving the conditioning of the matrix by choosing a measurement method for a resistivity distribution impedance is a very difficult task, since no explicit relationship can be seen. As an alternative, Hua *et al* (1988) used the regularization method to improve its conditioning.

10.10.1 The regularization method

In the regularization or Bayesian technique (Gottfried and Weisman 1973), the objective function to be minimized is

$$\Phi(\rho) = (1/2)(f(\rho) - V_0)^{T}(f(\rho) - V_0) + \lambda J(\rho). \tag{10.51}$$

The first term measures the fidelity to the measured data as in equation (10.36), while the second term, i.e., the penalty term, $J(\rho)$ takes the prior information into account. The smoothing parameter λ controls the relative weighting given to the prior information. In our application, we let $J(\rho)$ be a quadratic function of ρ, i.e., $J(\rho) = \rho^{T}\Sigma\rho$, where Σ is a positive-definite matrix, depending on the form of prior information we use. Thus the objective function is

$$\Phi(\rho) = (1/2)(f(\rho) - V_0)^{T}(f(\rho) - V_0) + \lambda\rho^{T}\Sigma\rho \tag{10.52}$$

The update procedure to search for the extremum of the above objective function can be shown to be

$$\rho^{k+1} = \rho^{k} + \Delta\rho^{k} \tag{10.53}$$

where

$$\Delta\rho^{k} = -[f'(\rho^{k})^{T}f'(\rho^{k}) + 2\lambda\Sigma]^{-1}[f'(\rho^{k})]^{T}[f(\rho^{k}) - V_0]. \tag{10.54}$$

Equation (10.54) differs from equation (10.42) only in the matrix to be inverted. Since Σ is a positive-definite matrix with λ nonnegative, the matrix to be inverted should have a better conditioning than that without regularization. In other words, the prior knowledge helps to stabilize the system.

10.10.2 The use of prior knowledge

In a practical problem, there is some prior information that we can use. If the solution is known to be bounded but fluctuating, we take the penalty form $J(\rho)$ as $||\rho||^2$; if the solution is continuous, then the penalty form $||\rho'||^2$, and if the solution is smooth, then $||\rho''||^2$.

In handling of the ill-conditioning, Murai and Kagawa (1985) used the SVD (Singular Value Decomposition) method, Akaike (1974) used the information criterion, and Yorkey *et al* (1986) used the Marquardt method (Marquardt 1963) because Bard (1970) showed that the Marquardt method performs better than the SVD and other methods. It can be shown that the Marquardt method is actually a regularization method corresponding to $J(\rho) = ||\rho||^2$, with the weighting coefficient λ adjusted at each iteration by the algorithm.

10.10.3 The choice of λ

The performance of the regularization method is closely related to the smoothing coefficient λ. A large λ distorts the information, while a small one has little effect. We are developing an algorithm which automatically determines a good coefficient depending on the experimental data.

10.10.4 Result

Figure 10.29 shows the reconstructed image using the Marquardt method with residual error 2.28, with the error being the normalized square error. Figures 10.30 and 10.31 use the $||\rho'||^2$, and $||\rho''||^2$ penalty forms with errors 0.447 and 0.444 respectively, with $\lambda = 0.001$. These images are much better than those of Marquardt. All the images are achieved after 20 iterations.

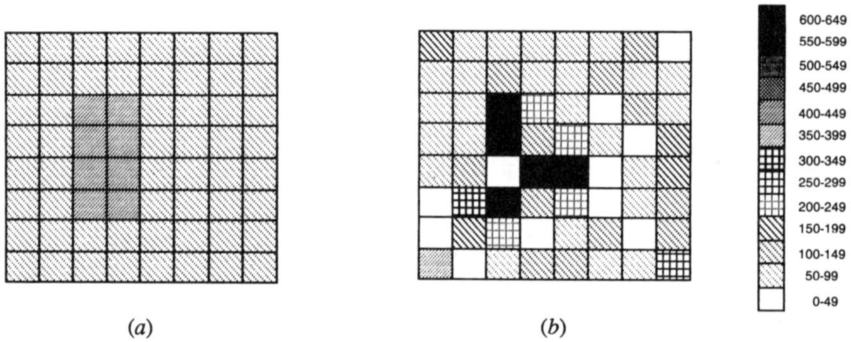

Figure 10.29 (*a*) The resistivity distribution to be reconstructed is an object of 350 Ω cm imbedded in a 75 Ω cm background. (*b*) The image reconstructed from data from (*a*) using the Marquardt method, which correspond to $J(\rho) = ||\rho||^2$.

10.11 SUMMARY OF EIT SYSTEMS

Table 10.1 is a summary of typical EIT systems developed by the University of Wisconsin–Madison, Rensselaer, Sheffield and Barcelona groups. It includes information about instruments, data collection methods and reconstruction algorithms. In table 10.1, unit time is the time for one voltage measurement and frame time is for all possible voltage measurements.

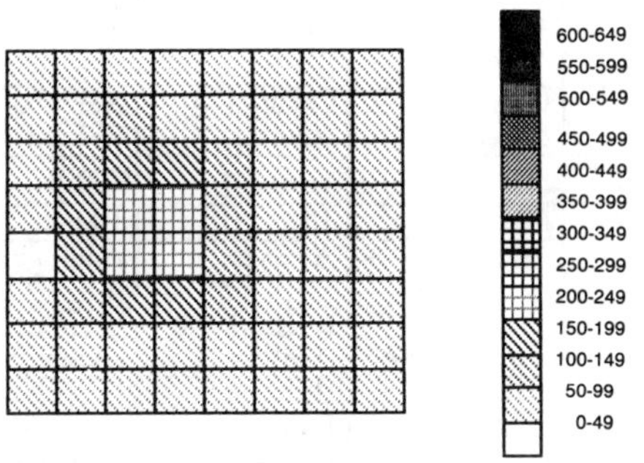

Figure 10.30 The image reconstructed from data from figure 10.29(*a*) using the penalty form $J(\rho) = \|\rho'\|^2$.

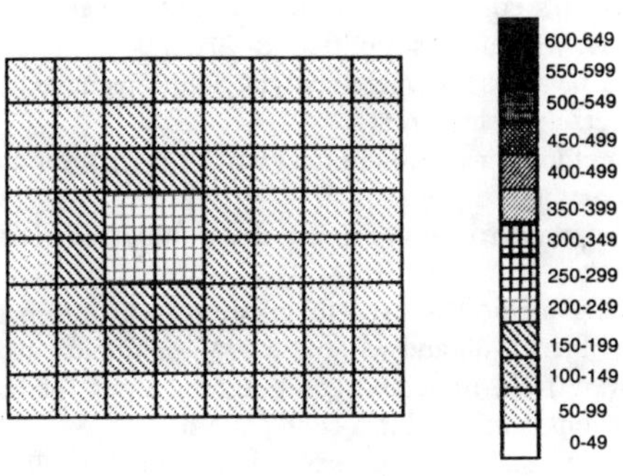

Figure 10.31 The image reconstructed from data from figure 10.29(*a*) using the penalty form $J(\rho) = \|\rho''\|^2$.

Table 10.1 Summary of typical EIT systems.

		Madison	Rensselaer	Sheffield	Barcelona
Data acquisition	Number of electrodes	32	32	16	16
	Frequency	50 kHz	15 kHz	50 kHz	10 – 100 kHz
	C. channel	32	32	1	1
	V. channel	1	1	1	16
	Accuracy	12 bit	12 bit	16 bit	16 bit
	2 or 4 electrode	4	2*	4	4
Data collection	Method	Optimal patterns	Optimal patterns	Neighboring method	Neighboring method
	Unit time	500 μs	16 ms	380 μs	400 μs
	Frame time	480 ms	15 s	100 ms	5.2 ms
Forward solution		FEM	Analytic	Analytic	Analytic
Inverse solution	Algorithm	N–R with regularization	N–R (single step)	Weighted backprojection	Weighted backprojection
	Iteration	10	1	1	1
Contact impedance		FEM	Lumped model	V not measured on I electrode	V not measured on I electrode
Image type		Static	Static	Dynamic	Dynamic
Spatial resolution	Simulation	10%	5%	10%	10 – 20%
	Phantom	10%	10%	10%	10 – 20%
	In vivo	Progress	10 – 20%	10 – 20%	10 – 20%

* They use all 32 electrodes to inject current and measure voltage.

10.12 STUDY QUESTIONS

10.1 Write the Poisson's equation, describe and define each operator and term in it and state how and why it can be simplified for EIT.

10.2 State and describe all cases where analytic solutions have been obtained for either the forward or inverse problem in EIT.

10.3 Describe the method for obtaining the element matrix for a quadrilateral element in a finite element method.

10.4 Describe the method for determining the number of elements to use in the finite element method.

10.5 The neighboring method is used to inject current into a two-dimensional circular homogeneous object with and without a center anomaly using eight equispaced point electrodes. Draw field lines and equipotential lines for both cases. Repeat for the cases when current is injected in a $\cos\theta$ pattern.

10.6 List the steps required in the backprojection method for EIT. Describe the advantages and disadvantages of this method.

10.7 List the steps required in the perturbation method for EIT. Why does the sensitivity matrix contain very different sensitivity values for the boundary and center areas? Describe the advantages and disadvantages of this method.

10.8 Describe the advantages and disadvantages of the applying-voltage-and-measuring-current method and injecting-current-and-measuring-voltage method.

10.9 List the steps required in the double constraint method for EIT. Describe the advantages and disadvantages of this method.

10.10 Using a simple sketch and equations, show how the Newton–Raphson method works for the one-dimensional case. Describe the advantages and disadvantages of this method.

10.11 Describe the necessary and sufficient conditions for the modified Newton–Raphson method to converge to a local minimum. Can you find the global minimum using the modified Newton–Raphson method? If so, under what conditions? If not, what is (are) the most important factors in helping it to find the global minimum?

10.12 What is the advantage of using the Hessian matrix in the modified Newton–Raphson method? Describe the steepest descent method and compare with the modified Newton–Raphson method.

10.13 Describe a single step algorithm which reconstructs difference EIT images using the Jacobian matrix in the Newton–Raphson method.

10.14 List the steps required in the sensitivity method for EIT.

10.15 Why and how is regularization used in EIT?

10.16 Define and explain ART.

10.17 Define and explain SIRT.

11

Computational Complexity

Eung Je Woo

In this chapter, we will discuss the amount of computation and storage needed for reconstruction algorithms described in Chapter 10. Since the repeated solution of the forward problem is required in reconstruction algorithms such as the modified Newton–Raphson and double constraint methods, we cover fast methods of solving the forward problem. Also, we discuss distributed and parallel implementations of the Newton–Raphson method.

11.1 FORWARD PROBLEM

11.1.1 Introduction

We describe the finite element method (FEM) as a numerical technique for solving the forward problem (equation (10.1)) for arbitrary conductivity distribution and boundary shape. Using the FEM, solving equation (10.1) results in solving a linear system of equations, equation (10.13). Therefore, first we discuss numerical techniques for solving a linear system of equations.

The method of solving a linear system of equations depends on the characteristics of the matrix. We observe that the matrix **Y** in equation (10.13) is symmetric, positive definite and very sparse (banded). Therefore, we are not concerned about the stability or ill-conditioning problem in solving equation (10.13). We focus only on the structure of **Y** matrix—not the numerical values of the matrix. Duff *et al* (1986) described various sparse matrix methods which take care of the stability and ill-conditioning problem using actual numerical values of a matrix.

In Chapter 10, we discussed two methods of solving a linear system of equations: the direct and the iterative methods. In EIT reconstruction algorithms, however, the direct method is advantageous since usually we need to solve a linear system of equations repeatedly with many right hand sides. Therefore, in this section, we focus on solving a sparse symmetric positive definite linear system of equations using direct methods (separate factorization and substitution). We will show later in this chapter that the iterative method is also used whenever it is advantageous in a reconstruction algorithm.

11.1.2 LU factorization

In order to solve a linear system of equations

$$\mathbf{Y}v = c \tag{11.1}$$

where $\mathbf{Y}$ is an $N \times N$ symmetric positive definite matrix, v is an unknown $N \times 1$ column vector, and c is a given $N \times 1$ column vector, we can express the matrix $\mathbf{Y}$ as a product of a lower and an upper triangular matrix, $\mathbf{L}$ and $\mathbf{U}$ by the LU Factorization (Conte and De Boor 1980, George and Liu 1981, Duff *et al* 1986). Since the $\mathbf{Y}$ matrix is symmetric, $\mathbf{U}$ is the transpose of $\mathbf{L}$ ($\mathbf{U} = \mathbf{L}^{\mathrm{T}}$). Then, the linear system of equations becomes

$$\mathbf{Y}v = \mathbf{L}\mathbf{L}^{\mathrm{T}}v = c. \tag{11.2}$$

Now let

$$\mathbf{L}^{\mathrm{T}}v = q \tag{11.3}$$

then,

$$\mathbf{L}q = c. \tag{11.4}$$

We first solve equation (11.4) for q by forward substitution, and then equation (11.3) for v by back substitution. The number of arithmetic operations involved in the factorization and substitution steps are $O(N^3/6)$ and $O(N^2)$, respectively. When we need to solve equation (11.1) with many right hand sides, we can repeat the forward/back substitution without factorizing the matrix again.

11.1.3 Structure of the Y matrix

Figure 11.1 shows the structure of the 389 × 389 $\mathbf{Y}$ matrix assembled from the mesh in figure 10.4 before and after factorization. In figure 11.1(*a*), we can see that the matrix $\mathbf{Y}$ is symmetric, banded and very sparse. Also the matrix is positive definite and usually diagonal dominant.

Figure 11.1(*b*) shows the structure of the $\mathbf{L} + \mathbf{U}$ matrix after the LU factorization of the matrix in figure 11.1(*a*). Since the matrix $\mathbf{Y}$ is very sparse, the LU factorization and forward/back substitution include many trivial computations such as multiplication by zero if we use a full matrix method. Also note that the LU factorization produces a large number of fill-ins which were zero in $\mathbf{Y}$ but are nonzero in $\mathbf{L}$ and $\mathbf{U}$. The number of fill-ins produced during LU factorization is determined by the way we number the nodes in the mesh. Changing the global node numbers in the mesh is equivalent to applying a permutation matrix to the assembled master matrix. Therefore, global node numbering determines the structure of the matrix $\mathbf{Y}$. And the number of fill-ins during LU factorization changes for different structures of the $\mathbf{Y}$ matrix.

11.2 SPARSE MATRIX METHOD

Based on observations about the characteristics of the $\mathbf{Y}$ matrix, we can reduce the computation time in solving equation (11.1) using sparse matrix methods.

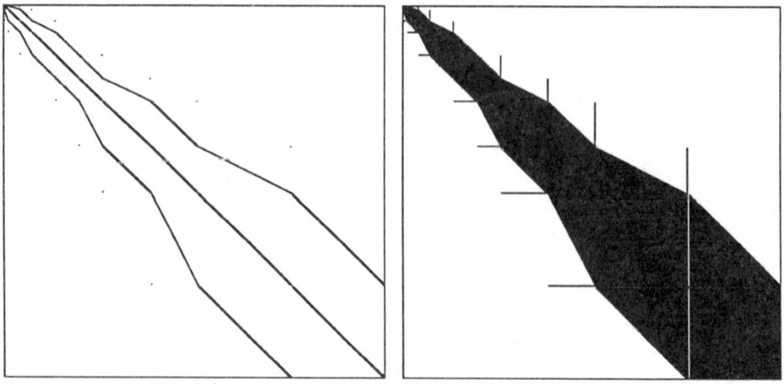

Figure 11.1 (*a*) Structure of the **Y** matrix (389 × 389) for the finite element mesh in figure 10.4. It has 2803 nonzero elements (1.85%). The global node numbers are assigned radially from the inside. (*b*) Structure of the **L** + **U** matrix after LU factorization of **Y**. It has 44849 nonzero elements (29.64%). Among them, 42046 elements (27.79%) are fill-ins.

There are many different sparse matrix techniques developed so far in the areas such as partial differential equations, power system analysis, electric circuit analysis, structural analysis, etc. The band matrix such as the one in figure 11.1(*a*) is typical of a matrix in structural analysis using the FEM. Matrices in power system analysis and electric circuit analysis do not usually have any special patterns. The band matrix can be considered as a special form of sparse matrix.

The basic idea of the sparse factorization and the sparse forward/back substitution routine is that we can avoid any trivial computations using the information about the matrix structure and a carefully designed data structure.

11.2.1 Analysis step

The analysis of a matrix structure is the first step in the sparse matrix method. The analysis step includes ordering (node renumbering) algorithms and symbolic factorization. Given a finite element mesh, we find a permutation vector using ordering algorithms which try to minimize the number of fill-ins during LU factorization. Then, the locations of all fill-ins in the factorized matrix are found by symbolic factorization.

Since the performance of most ordering algorithms depends on the matrix, we need to compare the performances of different ordering algorithms for a given sparse matrix (Duff *et al* 1986). In this chapter, we discuss six ordering algorithms: Tinney scheme 1, Tinney scheme 2, Tinney scheme 3, Cuthill–McKee, Reverse Cuthill–McKee and Gibbs–Poole–Stockmeyer. The first three are general methods for all types of sparse matrices and the last three are used only for band matrices.

Tinney scheme 1 (Sato and Tinney 1963, Duff et al 1986)

We define the valence of a row of a matrix as the number of nonzeros in the row. Since each row of the matrix corresponds to each node in the finite element mesh, the valence of a node can also be defined as the number of edges connected to the node in the corresponding graph of the finite element mesh. Tinney scheme 1 is known as '*a priori* ordering' and it orders rows (nodes) in the order of increasing valence without taking into account the fill-ins produced during LU factorization.

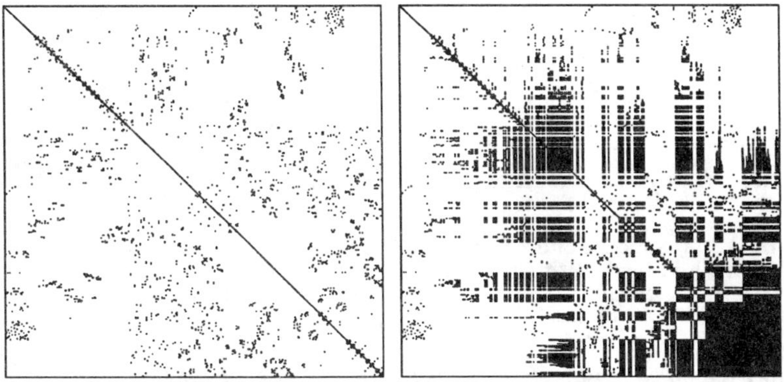

(*a*) (*b*)

Figure 11.2 (*a*) Structure of the **Y** matrix (389 × 389, 2803 nonzero elements) for the finite element mesh in figure 10.4 after Tinney scheme 1 ordering. (*b*) Structure of the **L** + **U** matrix after factorization. It has 29809 nonzero elements (19.70%). Among them, 27006 elements (17.85%) are fill-ins.

It is the fastest and simplest ordering method and gives satisfactory results when the total number of nodes (N) is relatively small (less than 100). However, the performance of this ordering method deteriorates for larger matrices. Figure 11.2(*a*) shows the structure of the **Y** matrix shown in figure 11.1(*a*) after using Tinney scheme 1 ordering and figure 11.2(*b*) shows the structure of the **L** + **U** matrix after factorization.

Tinney scheme 2 (Tinney and Walker 1967, Duff et al 1986)

Tinney scheme 2 is also called 'the minimum degree algorithm' or 'Markowitz ordering for symmetric matrix'. In this method, we generate a valence list and select the first pivot as a row (node) with the lowest valence (valence is defined as in the Tinney scheme 1). Then we eliminate this pivot and add all fill-ins caused by this elimination. We remove the pivotal row from the valence list and update the valences of rows which are affected by the elimination of the pivotal row. Now we select the next pivot as a row with the lowest valence in the current valence list. This procedure continues until the valence list is empty.

By using the permutation produced by the Tinney scheme 2, we could significantly reduce the number of fill-ins. This ordering algorithm has been proved to be the best for various kinds of symmetric sparse matrices in terms of performance and the needed computation time (Duff *et al* 1986, George and Liu 1981). Figure 11.3(*a*) shows the structure of the **Y** matrix shown in figure 11.1(*a*) after using the Tinney scheme 2 ordering and figure 11.3(*b*) is the structure of the **L** + **U** matrix after factorization.

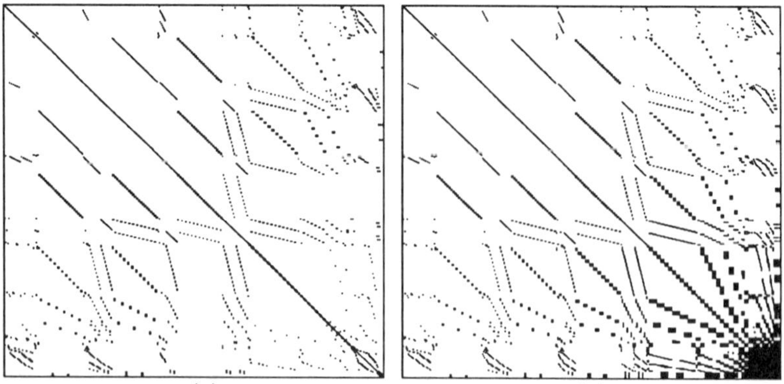

(*a*) (*b*)

Figure 11.3 (*a*) Structure of the **Y** matrix (389 × 389, 2803 nonzero elements) for the finite element mesh in figure 10.4 after Tinney scheme 2 ordering. (*b*) Structure of the **L** + **U** matrix after factorization. It has 7869 nonzero elements (5.20%). Among them, 5066 elements (3.35%) are fill-ins.

Tinney scheme 3 (Tinney and Walker 1967, Duff et al 1986)

Tinney scheme 3 is called 'the local minimum fill-in algorithm'. In this algorithm, we define the valence of a row as the number of fill-ins created if this row is eliminated at that stage of the LU factorization. In Tinney scheme 3, we simulate the elimination procedure for all rows and generate a valence list. We select the first pivot as the smallest valence row. Then, we eliminate this pivot and add all fill-ins caused by this elimination. We remove the pivotal row from the valence list and update the valences of rows which are affected by the elimination of the pivotal row. Now we select the next pivot as a row with the lowest valence in the current valence list. This procedure continues until the valence list is empty.

This method takes longer than Tinney scheme 2 since it requires simulated elimination steps. However, Tinney scheme 3 is not always better than Tinney scheme 2 in reducing the number of fill-ins produced during the LU factorization. Figure 11.4(*a*) shows the topology of the master matrix shown in figure 11.1 after using Tinney scheme 3 ordering and figure 11.4(*b*) is the topology of its **L** + **U** matrix.

Cuthill–McKee algorithm (Duff et al 1986, George and Liu 1981)

The Cuthill–McKee algorithm is an ordering algorithm for band matrices. The objective of this ordering algorithm is the minimization of the bandwidth of the matrix. Bandwidth B of a symmetrically structured matrix **A** is defined as

$$B = 2m + 1 \tag{11.5}$$

where m is the smallest integer such that $a_{ij} = 0$ whenever $|i - j| > m$. In this algorithm, we divide all nodes of a graph into level sets, S_i with S_1 consisting of a single arbitrary starting node. S_i $(i > 1)$ consists of all the ith neighbors of the starting node. Then, pivots are selected from $S_1, S_2, \ldots$, and S_D (D is the diameter of the graph).

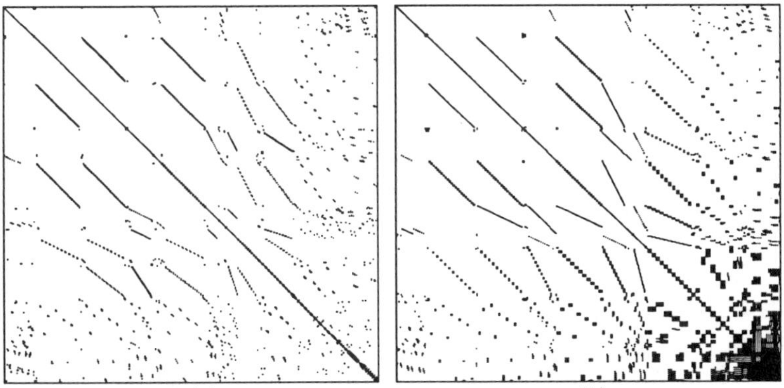

Figure 11.4 (*a*) Structure of the **Y** matrix (389 × 389, 2803 nonzero elements) for the finite element mesh in figure 10.4 after Tinney scheme 3 ordering. (*b*) Structure of the **L** + **U** matrix after factorization. It has 7693 nonzero elements (5.08%). Among them, 4890 elements (3.23%) are fill-ins.

Even though this ordering algorithm reduces the bandwidth of a matrix, it does not usually reduce the number of fill-ins during LU factorization compared with Tinney scheme 2 or 3. The performance of this ordering algorithm is highly dependent upon the selection of the starting node (Duff *et al* 1986).

Reverse Cuthill–McKee algorithm (Duff et al 1986, George and Liu 1981)
After using the Cuthill–McKee algorithm, we simply reverse the order. For certain types of matrices, the Reverse Cuthill–McKee algorithm is considerably better than the Cuthill–McKee algorithm. An important case is a finite element problem using elements with interior and edge nodes.

Gibbs–Poole–Stockmeyer algorithm (Gibbs et al 1976, Duff et al 1986, George and Liu 1981)
Gibbs *et al* (1976) select an arbitrary starting node and apply the Cuthill–McKee algorithm once. Then, they apply the Cuthill–McKee algorithm again using each node in the final level set S_D as a new starting node. If one of these nodes produces D' level sets and $D' > D$, then this node replaces the original starting node and all nodes in the level set $S_{D'}$ are tested again. Therefore, this algorithm tries to maximize the number of level sets by finding the best starting node for the Cuthill–McKee algorithm. This algorithm is considered to be the best for reducing the bandwidth.

Breaking ties
In all ordering algorithms, when more than one node has the same valence or is in the same level set, we select a node arbitrarily. However, there could be different permutation vectors depending on the way we select the pivot when this happens. Several tie-breaking algorithms have been developed, but none of them offers any significant improvement (Duff *et al* 1986).

Symbolic factorization

After we find a permutation vector using one of the above ordering algorithms, we can assemble the master matrix using the new global node numbers or permute the matrix already assembled. In the sparse matrix method, we store only nonzeros of the matrix. In order not to create a new storage area for a fill-in during the LU factorization, we find all fill-ins before the actual numerical LU factorization. This procedure is called symbolic factorization and the sparse matrix with all fill-ins added is called the perfect elimination matrix (Alvarado 1977).

11.2.2 Data structure

In implementing the sparse LU factorization and the sparse forward/back substitution routines, we need a special data structure to store the sparse matrix. Many different data structures have been suggested for different types of sparse matrices (Duff *et al* 1986, George and Liu 1981). The most used one in a general sparse matrix code is the row linked-list shown in figure 11.5. For band or variable-band matrices, simpler storage schemes can be used without any complicated data structure.

In the row linked-list data structure, we set up a linked-list for each row of the matrix. Therefore, there are total of N linked-lists and each of them contains all nonzero entries in the corresponding row of the perfect elimination matrix which includes all fill-ins.

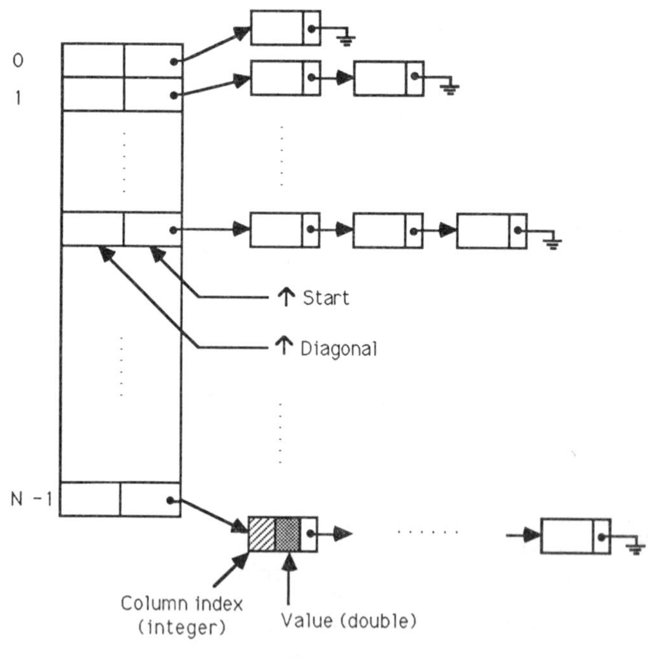

Figure 11.5 Row linked-list data structure.

11.2.3 Sparse LU factorization and substitution

Using the information about the matrix structure and the data structure in previous sections, we can implement a sparse LU factorization and a forward/back substitution routine. Let τ be the total number of nonzeros in a matrix, then for a sparse matrix

$$\tau = O(N^{1+\gamma}) \tag{11.6}$$

where N is the dimension of the matrix and $\gamma < 1$. Then, the number of arithmetic operations involved in the sparse factorization and substitution step could be $O(N^{1+2\gamma})$ and $O(N^{1+\gamma})$, respectively. Therefore, we can reduce the computation time significantly by a careful implementation of sparse factorization and substitution routines.

11.2.4 Storage requirement for the forward problem

The amount of memory needed for storing the **Y** matrix depends on the data structure used and the number of bytes used in representing a real number. Let the total number of nonzeros in the **L** + **U** matrix (or in the perfect elimination matrix) be τ and assume that we use the data structure shown in figure 11.5, then we need

$$S_Y = \tau \times (B_I + B_R + B_P) \tag{11.7}$$

bytes of memory where B_I, B_R and B_P are the number of bytes used for representing integers, real numbers and pointers (address).

Assuming that $B_I = 2$, $B_R = 12$ and $B_P = 4$, for the matrix shown in figure 11.3(*b*), $S_Y = 7869 \times (2 + 12 + 4) = 141642$ bytes (≈138.4 kbyte). If we use a full matrix method and store the **Y** matrix in a two-dimensional array, we need $389 \times 389 \times 12 = 1815852$ bytes (≈1.74 Mbyte) of memory. Therefore, we can significantly reduce not only the computation time but also the memory by using sparse matrix techniques. We also need memory for storing vectors $\boldsymbol{c}$ and $\boldsymbol{v}$. However, even though we need to solve equation (11.1) for many $\boldsymbol{c}$'s and $\boldsymbol{v}$'s, the total storage requirement for these vectors is usually less than 10 kbyte.

11.2.5 Example

Figure 11.6 shows three finite element meshes used to test the sparse matrix method. Figure 11.6 (*c*) is the same as the mesh in figure 10.4.

Table 11.1 shows the required computation times for solving three linear systems of equations corresponding to three meshes in figure 11.6 using full matrix methods and iterative methods. In table 11.1 Gaussian denotes the Gaussian elimination and Cholesky denotes the Cholesky factorization with forward/back substitution. C.G.* denotes the conjugate gradient method where we stop the iteration when the error difference < 0.000244. In implementing the sparse conjugate gradient method (C.G.**), we take full advantage of the sparsity of the matrix and avoid any trivial computations in the routine where we multiply the matrix by a vector.

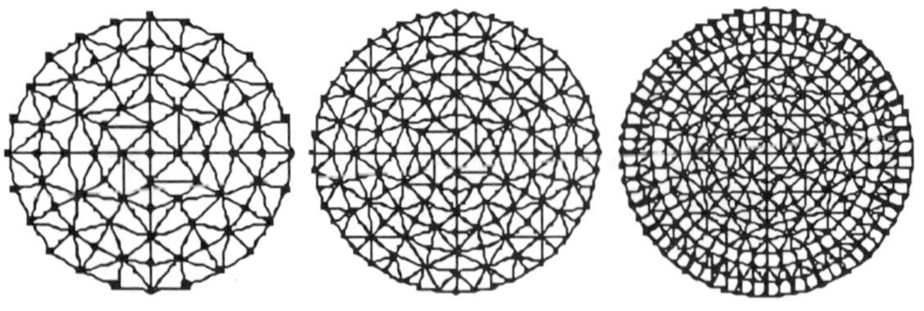

(a) (b) (c)

Model	N	T	R	E	Spatial resolution(%)
(a)	77	128	80 – 128	– 24	10
(b)	149	248	128 – 248	– 48	7
(c)	389	536	256 – 536	– 96	5

(d)

Figure 11.6 (a) – (c) Three different sizes of finite element meshes. (d) Specifications of each model. N is the number of nodes, T is the number of elements, R is the number of resistivity values to be determined by the reconstruction algorithm and E is the number of nodes on the boundary. R changes depending on how we group the elements.

Table 11.1 Computation times in seconds for solving a 77×77, 149×149 and 389×389 linear system of equations. F denotes factorization and S denotes forward/back substitution. All tests were performed on a Macintosh II.

Model	Method			
	Gaussian (s)	Cholesky (s)	C.G.* (s)	C.G.** (s)
77×77	6.83	F: 1.65 S: 0.17	4.70	1.52
149×149	49.30	F: 11.65 S: 0.60	21.82	4.15
389×389	877.97	F: 201.90 S: 4.07	295.38	24.15

* Conjugate gradient method without taking advantage of sparsity
** Sparse conjugate gradient method

Table 11.2 shows the performance of three ordering algorithms: Tinney scheme 1, 2 and 3 for three meshes in figure 11.6. Compared to the results in table 11.1, the sparse matrix method significantly reduces the computation times. Table 11.1 shows that the amount of computation time for the factorization increases with the cube of the number of nodes ($\sim O(N^3)$). However, in table 11.2, the computation time increases less than the square of the number of nodes ($\sim O(N^{1.85})$) due to the sparse matrix method. Therefore, there is a greater reduction in the computation time for larger models.

Table 11.2 also shows that the application of the ordering algorithm could provide a maximal reduction to 1/32 of the computation time compared to the case when we do not use any ordering algorithm. In table 11.2, the Tinney scheme 3 algorithm produces the smallest number of fill-ins even though there is not a big difference between the Tinney scheme 3 and scheme 2. However, if the computation time for the Tinney scheme 3 or the difference between the Tinney scheme 3 and scheme 2 does not justify its use, the Tinney scheme 2 is a good choice since it is fast and also almost as efficient as Tinney scheme 3.

Table 11.2 Computation times in seconds for the sparse matrix method with/without ordering algorithms. F denotes factorization and S denotes forward/back substitution. All tests were performed on a Macintosh II.

Model	Scheme	Fill-ins	Solver 1* (s)		Solver 2** (s)	
			F	S	F	S
77 × 77	None	2106(35.52%)	0.78	0.07	1.22	0.07
	Scheme1	952(16.06%)	0.33	0.05	0.62	0.05
	Scheme2	438(7.39%)	0.12	0.02	0.25	0.02
	Scheme3	414(6.98%)	0.10	0.02	0.23	0.02
149 × 149	None	6392(28.79%)	3.23	0.22	5.05	0.20
	Scheme1	2520(11.35%)	1.03	0.10	2.18	0.10
	Scheme2	1174(5.29%)	0.32	0.08	0.82	0.07
	Scheme3	1174(5.29%)	0.32	0.08	0.82	0.07
389 × 389	None	42046(27.79%)	54.25	1.33	78.18	1.15
	Scheme1	27006(17.85%)	33.43	0.92	57.28	0.78
	Scheme2	5066(3.35%)	1.80	0.25	4.90	0.22
	Scheme3	4890(3.23%)	1.68	0.23	4.48	0.22

* LU factorization using row linked-list
** Cholesky factorization using packed linear array

11.2.6 Discussion

A fast algorithm for solving the forward problem is very important when reconstructing static images using the iterative equipotential lines method, modified Newton–Raphson method or double constraint method. Since the FEM is mostly used in solving the forward problem, we introduce sparse matrix techniques for solving a linear system of equations. Further reduction in computation time is also possible by using sparse vector methods (Tinney *et al* 1985). Since the right hand side $\boldsymbol{c}$ in equation (11.1) is a sparse vector and we only need to compute a small number of elements in $\boldsymbol{v}$ (only boundary node voltages), sparse vector methods can be used in EIT.

Instead of the general sparse matrix methods discussed here, band or variable-band (profile) methods could be used in EIT since the $\mathbf{Y}$ matrix is banded. For band methods, the Gibbs–Poole–Stockmeyer ordering algorithm is useful in reducing the bandwidth. Band methods are easier to implement but general sparse matrix methods using row linked-list data structures provide better performance in reducing the amount of computation. Also the general method can more easily adapted to the sparse vector method for further reduction in computation time.

In order to solve forward problems repeatedly in image reconstruction, the sparse matrix methods described here or any other efficient methods of solving equation (11.1) are essential in reducing both the computation time and storage requirement.

11.3 BACKPROJECTION METHOD

The noniterative backprojection between equipotential lines method does not need the solution of the forward problem during image reconstruction. Since the computation of the equipotential lines is done before the image reconstruction, this method is very fast and does not need a large storage area.

However, iterative methods require a solution of the forward problem for each iteration to compute new equipotential lines. Therefore, the computation time for image reconstruction is highly dependent on the computation time for solving the forward problem. Also, the storage requirement for the **Y** matrix dominates the total storage requirements.

11.4 DOUBLE CONSTRAINT METHOD

The double constraint method described in Chapter 10 also requires solution of the forward problem twice in each iteration. Since the amount of computation involved in equation (10.33) is relatively small, the computation time for image reconstruction is highly dependent on the computation time for solving the forward problem. Also, the storage requirement for the **Y** matrix dominates the total storage requirements. Compared to the iterative backprojection method in the previous section, the double constraint method requires approximately twice the computation time (Yorkey *et al* 1987a).

11.5 MODIFIED NEWTON–RAPHSON METHOD

The modified Newton–Raphson method is described in Section 10.7. This method is known to be the most sophisticated one and there are several different ways of implementing this method. Here, we discuss various computational aspects of the method including computation of the objective function, Jacobian matrix, Hessian matrix and update of the resistivity distribution.

11.5.1 Computation of the objective function

Let ρ be the R-dimensional vector corresponding to the discrete resistivity distribution. Let v_0 be the M-dimensional voltage vector whose elements are the voltages we measure from the surface of an object due to injection currents and f be a function from an R-dimensional resistivity distribution vector into a M-dimensional voltage vector. $f(\rho)$ is calculated using the FEM for the same injection current and the same electrode configuration we use for the measurement of v_0. Then, in Chapter 10, the objective function $\Phi(\rho)$ was defined as the squared error difference between the measured and calculated voltage responses.

$$\Phi(\rho) = \frac{1}{2}(f(\rho) - v_0)^{\mathrm{T}}(f(\rho) - v_0). \tag{11.8}$$

To obtain a complete voltage measurement set, we need to inject more than one distribution of current. Define a single distribution of injection current as a projection, and let the number of projections be P. Then, we need to solve the following linear system of equations to compute $f(\rho)$:

$$\mathbf{YV} = \mathbf{C} \tag{11.9}$$

where $\mathbf{Y}$ is the $N \times N$ matrix (N is the number of nodes in the mesh), $\mathbf{V} = [v_1, v_2, \ldots, v_P]$ is the $N \times P$ node voltage matrix, and $\mathbf{C} = [c_1, c_2, \ldots, c_P]$ is the $N \times P$ node current matrix. Actually, we solve the linear system of equations P times for each v_i with each c_i. From the $N \times P$ matrix $\mathbf{V}$, we can form a $NP \times 1$ vector by stacking all columns of $\mathbf{V}$ as described in Chapter 10. Now we define vec($\mathbf{V}$) as follows:

$$\mathrm{vec}(\mathbf{V}) = [v_1^{\mathrm{T}}, v_2^{\mathrm{T}}, \ldots, v_P^{\mathrm{T}}]^{\mathrm{T}}. \tag{11.10}$$

Since vec($\mathbf{V}$) contains all the node voltages including internal nodes for all projections, we must extract node voltages corresponding to the voltage measuring electrodes. Define a $M \times NP$ matrix $\mathbf{T}$ as a transformation matrix which extracts those node voltages from vec($\mathbf{V}$). Then,

$$f(\rho) = \mathbf{T}\mathrm{vec}(\mathbf{V}). \tag{11.11}$$

We use sparse matrix methods described in the previous section to solve equation (11.9) for $\mathbf{V}$. The amount of computation for $f(\rho)$ is, therefore, P times that required for the solution of the linear system of equations.

11.5.2 Calculation of the Jacobian matrix

The Jacobian matrix $\mathbf{J}$ ($M \times R$) is

$$\mathbf{J} = f'(\rho) = \mathbf{T}\mathrm{vec}(\mathbf{V})' = \mathbf{T}\mathrm{vec}(\mathbf{Y}^{-1}\mathbf{C})' = \mathbf{TQ} \tag{11.12}$$

where $\mathbf{Q}$ is an $NP \times R$ partitioned matrix, where the (i, j)th partition q_{ij} is

$$q_{ij} = \frac{\partial \mathbf{Y}^{-1}}{\partial \rho_j} c_i = -\mathbf{Y}^{-1}\frac{\partial \mathbf{Y}}{\partial \rho_j}\mathbf{Y}^{-1}c_i = -\mathbf{Y}^{-1}\frac{\partial \mathbf{Y}}{\partial \rho_j} v_i. \tag{11.13}$$

Therefore, as shown in figure 11.7, there are PR partitions, and each partition ($N \times 1$ vector) is calculated by solving the following linear system of equations:

$$\mathbf{Y}q_{ij} = \frac{\partial \mathbf{Y}}{\partial \rho_j} v_i. \tag{11.14}$$

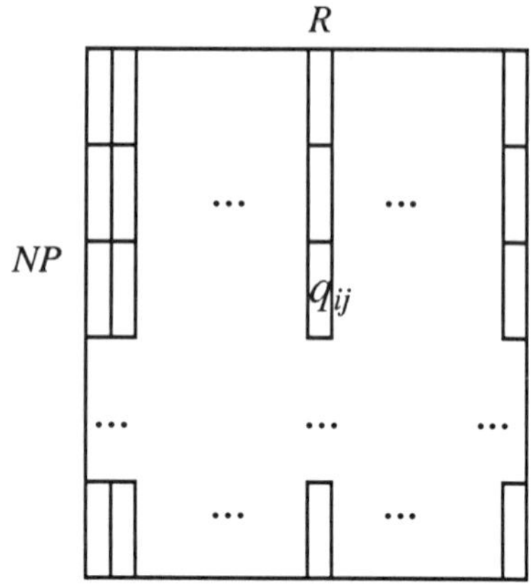

Figure 11.7 Partitioned **Q** matrix

Note that the matrix **Y** in equation (11.14) is the same as the matrix in equation (11.9). Therefore, for a given resistivity distribution, we assemble the matrix **Y** and perform the sparse LU factorization just once. Then, we solve both equations (11.9) and (11.14) by repeated application of the sparse forward/back substitutions. The amount of computation for the matrix **J** is *PR* times that required for the solution of the linear system of equations.

11.5.3 Calculation of resistivity update

In Chapter 10, the resistivity update in each iteration is shown in equation (10.40). However, the resistivity update, $\Delta\rho^k$ is actually calculated by solving the following linear system of equations:

$$[f'(\rho^k)^{\mathrm{T}} f'(\rho^k)]\,\Delta\rho^k = -f'(\rho^k)^{\mathrm{T}}\,(f(\rho^k) - v_0). \tag{11.15}$$

Now we discuss different methods of computing the resistivity update.

Conventional method (method 1)
Solving equation (11.15) for $\Delta\rho^k$ requires three steps. First, we need to compute the approximate Hessian matrix **H** ($R \times R$),

$$\mathbf{H} = f'(\rho^k)^{\mathrm{T}} f'(\rho^k). \tag{11.16}$$

The second step is the multiplication of the matrix $f'(\rho^k)^{\mathrm{T}}$ by the vector $(f(\rho^k) - v_0)$. Let

$$p = -f'(\rho^k)^{\mathrm{T}}\,(f(\rho^k) - v_0). \tag{11.17}$$

Then, we need to solve the following linear system of equations for $\Delta\rho^k$:

$$\mathbf{H}\Delta\rho^k = p. \tag{11.18}$$

We can use either a direct method or an iterative method to solve equation (11.18). However, since it is known that $\mathbf{H}$ is ill-conditioned, the computed solution $\Delta\rho^k$ is very sensitive to errors in $\mathbf{H}$ and p including round off, measurement and finite element modeling error. Therefore, in Chapter 10, the regularized method is described to overcome the ill-conditioning problem. Iterative refinement can also be used to improve the accuracy of the solution (Conte and De Boor 1980, Duff *et al* 1986). In the following section, we discuss different numerical techniques for solving equation (11.15).

Hachtel's method (method 2)
Gjelsvik *et al* (1985) used Hachtel's augmented matrix method in power system static state estimation to improve numerical stability. The same technique can be used with the modified Newton–Raphson method. Equation (11.15) can be rewritten as follows:

$$[\mathbf{J}^{\mathrm{T}}\mathbf{J}]\Delta\rho^k = \mathbf{J}^{\mathrm{T}}b \tag{11.19}$$

where $b = -(f(\rho^k) - v_0)$.

Instead of computing the matrix multiplication $\mathbf{J}^{\mathrm{T}}\mathbf{J}$ and solving the $R \times R$ linear system of equations, we can formulate a new linear system of equations with an augmented sparse $(R + M) \times (R + M)$ matrix as follows:

$$\begin{bmatrix} \mathbf{I} & \mathbf{J} \\ \mathbf{J}^{\mathrm{T}} & \mathbf{0} \end{bmatrix} \begin{bmatrix} r \\ \Delta\rho^k \end{bmatrix} = \begin{bmatrix} b \\ 0 \end{bmatrix}. \tag{11.20}$$

When the condition number of $\mathbf{J}$ is κ, the condition number of $\mathbf{J}^{\mathrm{T}}\mathbf{J}$ is κ^2. Therefore, matrix multiplication makes the conditioning of the linear system of equations (11.18) worse. By solving equation (11.20) instead of equations (11.16), (11.17) and (11.18), we can avoid making the conditioning worse. This method is also advantageous because it reduces computation. First, we do not need to compute $\mathbf{J}^{\mathrm{T}}\mathbf{J}$ which takes about 25% of the total computation time of the modified Newton–Raphson method (see Section 11.5.6). Second, even though the new linear system of equations is larger, we can take advantage of the sparsity of the augmented matrix. Also in solving equation (11.20) for $\Delta\rho^k$, it is better to use iterative methods such as SOR and the conjugate gradient method since they could be faster than direct methods and also easily parallelizable (see Section 11.5.8).

QR factorization method (method 3)
Equation (11.15) is of the same form as the normal equation in least squares. Hager (1988) describes the solution of the normal equation using QR factorization. Since QR factorization is numerically much more stable than LU factorization, this method could be better in solving such an ill-conditioned linear system of equations.

11.5.4 Storage requirement

The amount of memory needed for storing the master matrix **Y** dominates the total storage requirement of reconstruction algorithms such as the iterative equipotential lines method and the double constraint method. In the modified Newton–Raphson method, in addition to this storage requirement, we need more memory for the Jacobian matrix **J** in equation (11.12) and the Hessian matrix **H** in equation (11.16). Since these matrices are dense, we use two-dimensional arrays. The $M \times R$ **J** matrix needs

$$S_J = M \times R \times B_R \tag{11.21}$$

bytes of memory. The $R \times R$ **H** matrix needs

$$S_H = R \times R \times B_R \tag{11.22}$$

bytes of memory. When $M = E \times P = 32 \times 8 = 256$, $R = 200$ and $B_R = 12$, $S_J =$ 614 400 bytes (600 kbyte) and $S_H = 480\,000$ bytes (468.75 kbyte).

We also needed about 138.4 kbytes for storing the **Y** matrix shown in figure 11.3(b) using the row linked-list. Therefore, the total minimal memory requirement for reconstructing the resistivity image using the mesh in figure 10.4 and given values of M and R is more than 1 Mbyte. In practice, we need more memory for storing other various information and the actual storage requirement varies depending upon the detail of the implementation. Therefore, the total storage requirement for the modified Newton–Raphson method, S_{NR} is

$$S_{NR} > S_Y + S_J + S_H. \tag{11.23}$$

11.5.5 Numerical experience

Table 11.3 shows the computation times of four parts of the reconstruction program for the three different sizes of models in figure 11.6(a), (b) and (c). OPCD is the computation time for calculating P optimal patterns of injection currents as described in Chapter 8. JACOB is the computation time for computing the Jacobian matrix. HESSN is the computation time for computing the approximate Hessian matrix by matrix multiplication. UPDAT is the computation time for solving equation (11.18) by Gaussian elimination with scaled partial column pivoting.

Assuming that 10 iterations of the modified Newton–Raphson method are required to reconstruct a resistivity image, we need 20 min 54 s, 40 min 24 s and 4 h 18 min 12 s to achieve about 10%, 7% and 5% spatial resolution, respectively. For a complicated resistivity distribution, we might need more than eight projections, then the computation time would increase. N, R, E and P are important factors in determining accuracy of the solution of the forward problem, the spatial resolution and also the computational complexity.

11.5.6 Limitation of algorithmic approach

As shown in table 11.3, there is a limit in reducing the computation time using an algorithmic approach on a single processor. If we increase the number of

Table 11.3 The last column is the minimal computation time of one iteration in minutes. Model (*a*), (*b*) and (*c*) are shown in figure 11.6(*a*), (*b*) and (*c*), respectively. *N* is the number of nodes, *P* is the number of projections, *E* is the number of electrodes and *R* is the number of resistivity values to be determined by the reconstruction algorithm. All tests were performed on a Macintosh II.

Model	OPCD (m)	JACOB (m)	HESSN (m)	UPDAT (m)	Iteration (m)
(*a*)*	1.12	0.35	0.47	0.15	2.09
(*b*)**	1.78	1.22	1.17	0.57	4.74
(*c*)***	7.17	8.00	6.23	4.42	25.82

* *N* is 77, *P* is 8, *E* is 24 and *R* is 80
** *N* is 77, *P* is 8, *E* is 24 and *R* is 128
*** *N* is 389, *P* is 8, *E* is 32 and *R* is 256

electrodes or implement a three-dimensional image reconstruction algorithm, the increase in computation time makes the EIT system impractical. Two approaches to overcome this problem have been tried. One method is to use a much more powerful remote computer through a network. The other is to use add-on parallel processor boards on a personal computer used in current EIT systems.

11.5.7 Distributed computation

Goble and Gallagher (1988) implemented the modified Newton–Raphson method on a Sun 3/60 workstation, Sun 4/280, IBM 3081-D and Cray X-MP/48. For a 32-electrode EIT system with a 496-element mesh, the run times of a single iteration on each machine are shown in table 11.4.

Table 11.4 Run times of a single iteration of the modified Newton–Raphson method (Goble and Gallagher 1988).

Computer	Run time (seconds)
Sun 3/60 workstation	3239
Sun 4/280	350
IBM 3081-D	165
Cray X-MP/48	6

They used an IBM PC-AT for data collection. Local hardware components were connected through a baseband Ethernet and had access to other computers via the broadband network on campus. The Cray X-MP located at the Pittsburgh Supercomputing Center was also accessed through a network. For the display, they used an IBM PC/XT-286 in the lab. Therefore, their distributed EIT system consisted of three computers connected through a network, one for data collection, one for image reconstruction and one for display.

This distributed approach made it possible for a single EIT system to share and utilize powerful remote computing resources. However, it also made it hard to design an inexpensive portable EIT system.

11.5.8 Parallel computation

Since many add-on parallel processor boards for a personal computer are available, parallelizing the reconstruction algorithm might be a better solution.

Parallelization

The computation of the objective function and Jacobian matrix requires a repeated solution of the same linear system of equations containing many right hand sides. Therefore, multiple processors could perform the forward/back substitution simultaneously on different right hand sides. By evenly distributing the total work to n processors, we could achieve a maximal $1/n$ reduction in computation time.

The computation of the $\mathbf{H}$ matrix in method 1 of Section 11.5.3 is a simple matrix multiplication which is very easily parallelizable. However, if we use a direct method of solving equation (11.18), this step would not be easily parallelizable unless we used R processors (Bertsekas and Tsitsiklis 1989). If we used method 2 and solved equation (11.20) using an iterative method such as SOR or the conjugate gradient method, we could easily parallelize the computation of the resistivity update without explicitly computing the $\mathbf{H}$ matrix.

Implementation on the Symmetry

The modified Newton–Raphson algorithm was implemented on a parallel computer system, the Symmetry from Sequent Computer Systems, Inc. The Symmetry system has 20 processors with 256 Mbyte of virtual address space per processor. All processors are tightly coupled and can access shared data structure in memory. The results shown in the following section were obtained using Sequent C language on the DYNIX operating system (Sequent Computer Systems Inc. 1987).

Results

Figure 11.8 shows the reduction in computation times for the conventional method (method 1). In figure 11.8, N is 37, E is 16, R is 56 and P is 8. GE is the computation time for solving equation (11.18) using the Gaussian elimination with scaled partial pivoting. GE does not change with the number of processors because it is not parallelized. H is the computation time for calculating the $\mathbf{H}$ matrix in equation (11.16). J is the computation time for computing the $\mathbf{J}$ matrix in equation (11.12). Total is the total computation time of a single iteration of the reconstruction algorithm.

Figure 11.9 shows the reduction in computation times for Hachtel's method (method 2). In figure 11.9, the size of the problem is exactly the same as figure 11.8. CG is the computation time for solving equation (11.20) using the parallelized conjugate gradient method and J is the computation time for computing the $\mathbf{J}$ matrix in equation (11.12). Total is the total computation time of a single iteration of the reconstruction algorithm.

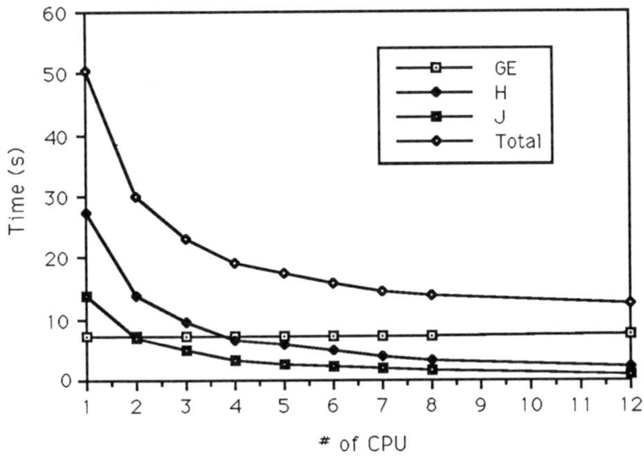

Figure 11.8 Computation times of a single iteration of the modified Newton–Raphson method using method 1 in Section 11.5.3 for the resistivity update calculation.

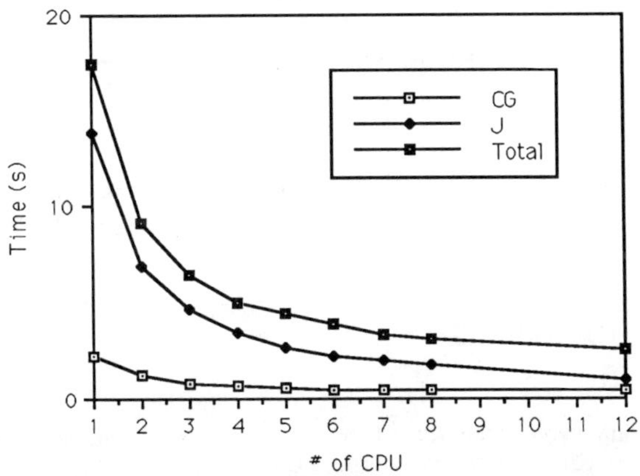

Figure 11.9 Computation times for a single iteration of the modified Newton–Raphson method using method 2 in Section 11.5.3 for the resistivity update calculation.

Figure 11.10 shows the reduction in computation time with the number of processors using Hachtel's method for a larger problem. In figure 11.10, N is 141, E is 32, R is 248 and P is 8.

Discussion

The increase in N will not increase the overall computation time significantly because we use sparse matrix methods. In Hachtel's method, we spend most of the computation time in calculating the Jacobian matrix **J**. Since this requires the solution of a $N \times N$ linear system of equations PR times, an increase in P or R requires a larger amount of computation. In practice, the maximal value of P

is given by $E/2$ and E is determined by the instrument ($E = 16$ or 32 in the current instruments). Also, the number R which can be determined by the reconstruction algorithm is given by $R < E(E-1)/2$ (see Chapter 10). However, the practical maximal value of R for a 32-electrode system ($E = 32$) is about 150 due to the nonlinearity of the problem and weak sensitivity of the center area. Therefore, figure 11.10 provides enough practical information about how much we can reduce the computation time for the current EIT system using parallel algorithms and a parallel computer.

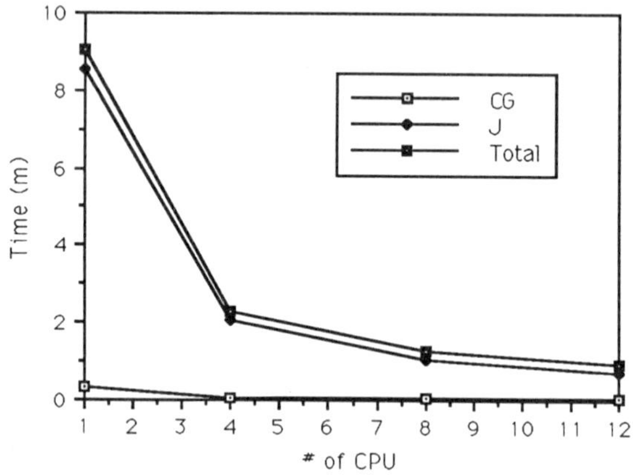

Figure 11.10 Computation times for a single iteration of the modified Newton–Raphson method using method 1 in section 11.5.3 for the resistivity update calculation for $N = 141$, $E = 32$, $R = 248$ and $P = 8$.

11.6 STUDY QUESTIONS

11.1 Write a computer program for LU factorization. Use the minimal amount of memory.

11.2 Explain why fill-ins are created during LU factorization.

11.3 Under what condition does the iterative method of solving equation (11.1) converge?

11.4 What is a positive definite matrix? Why is the master matrix from the FEM positive definite? Describe the Cholesky factorization algorithm.

11.5 Describe the physical reason why the matrix in figure 11.1(a) is very sparse.

11.6 Describe the Tinney scheme 2 matrix ordering algorithm.

11.7 Describe three steps in solving equation (11.1) using sparse matrix methods.

11.8 What is ill-conditioning? What could happen in the solution of a linear system of equations with a ill-conditioned matrix? Why is the Hessian matrix in the modified Newton–Raphson method ill-conditioned?

11.9 Define the condition number of a square matrix. Define the condition number of matrix **J** in equation (11.12) (note that **J** is not a square matrix). What is the condition number of the **H** matrix? What is the condition number of the augmented matrix in equation (11.20)?

11.10 When equation (11.1) is solved using a direct method, the solution may not be correct due to the ill-conditioning of the matrix. Describe methods of improving the accuracy of the solution.

11.11 Compare the number of computations for the backprojection, double constraint and Newton–Raphson methods.

11.12 Compare the amount of storage for the backprojection, double constraint and Newton–Raphson methods.

11.13 You decided to implement the modified Newton–Raphson method on a parallel computer system with 20 processors. How would you distribute the total work (computational load) to 20 processors? What kind of parallel computer system would you use?

11.14 Describe the advantages and disadvantages of the distributed and parallel computations in EIT image reconstruction.

12

Measures of Performance

Mark Heimbach

The purpose of noninvasive EIT systems is to visualize internal regions of the human body by means of external electrodes. Due to varying resistivities of internal organs, current passed through the body results in voltage changes measured on the surface. The performance of an EIT system can be stated in terms of spatial resolution, conductivity resolution, conductivity contrast and some other parameters described in this chapter. We will define these terms and discuss various design factors related to them.

12.1 INTRODUCTION

An objective in EIT imaging is to maximize the boundary voltage change due to an anomaly so it is more readily seen in relation to its background. Two measures related to the magnitude of this change in surface potential are the anomaly's size and resistivity compared to the assumed size and resistivity of the surrounding body. Figure 12.1(*a*) shows a circular object with a circular anomaly at the center. Using the model in figure 12.1(*a*), Seagar and Bates (1985) derived and experimentally verified the equations relating the image quality parameters with the system design factors for the two current sources and many voltage measurements configuration. Seagar *et al* (1987) also derived similar equations for the many current sources and many voltage measurements configuration with the same model. In the former case, the location of the two current injection electrodes becomes one of the important parameters. However, it has been shown that injecting patterns of current using many current sources provides better performance (Isaacson 1986, Gisser *et al* 1987). An object with an offset anomaly in figure 12.1(*b*) can also be analyzed in the same way by a conformal transformation between figures 12.1(*a*) and (*b*).

Seagar *et al* (1987) defined three parameters. First, the spatial resolution is defined as the smallest region of a medium into which the conductivity can be independently determined. In figure 12.1,

$$\text{Spatial resolution} = \frac{r_a}{r_b}. \tag{12.1}$$

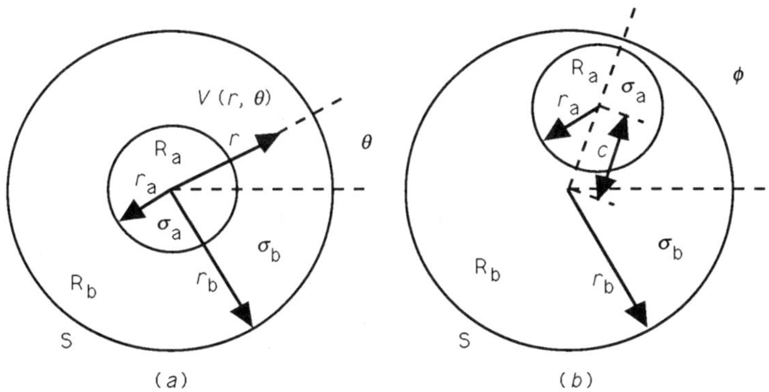

Figure 12.1 Circular objects with (*a*) a center anomaly and (*b*) an offset anomaly.

The spatial resolution is then the degree to which nearly equal conductivities of two objects can be discriminated. Second, the conductivity contrast is the ratio between the conductivity of an anomaly to that of its surrounding region. In figure 12.1,

$$\text{Conductivity contrast} = \alpha = \frac{\sigma_a}{\sigma_b}. \tag{12.2}$$

Third, the conductivity resolution is now defined as the fractional change in conductivity contrast. Therefore,

$$\text{Conductivity resolution} = \frac{\delta\alpha}{\alpha}. \tag{12.3}$$

Limits of the spatial and conductivity resolution are mainly determined by measurement errors such as quantization errors, movement artifacts and electrode location errors. A further error is introduced by the reconstruction algorithm used. In this chapter, however, we do not include errors caused by reconstruction algorithms in the analysis.

Changes in tissue conductivity can only be resolved if measurement errors are less than the difference between the measured boundary voltage from an object with an anomaly and the boundary voltage from a homogeneous body. The fractional change in the boundary voltage ($\delta V/V$) is, therefore, considered to be equal to the measurement error or noise in the analysis in Sections 12.2 and 12.3.

In Section 12.4, the concept of distinguishability is introduced to provide the optimal method for locating interior objects so that maximal current can be passed through that area. Finally, methods for imaging moving objects within the body will be discussed in Section 12.5.

12.2 VISIBILITY AND SENSITIVITY

12.2.1 Selection of injection currents and driving point impedance

In order to maximize the voltage changes at the surface electrodes, injected current must be targeted to regions where an anomaly is assumed to be located. For the object in figure 12.1(*a*), Isaacson (1986) and Gisser *et al* (1987) proved that the following is the optimal pattern of injection currents in terms of maximizing the distinguishability (see Sections 8.6 and 12.4). That is, the optimal injection currents produce the maximal difference between the boundary voltages measured from the object in figure 12.1(*a*) and from the object without any anomaly (homogeneous). Let $J_n(\theta)$ be the optimal current density distributions impressed on the boundary, then

$$J_n(\theta) = A_n \cos n\theta + B_n \sin n\theta \quad (n = 1, 2, ...) \tag{12.4}$$

where $n = 1$ is the best injection current since it produces the maximal distinguishability. The distinguishability decreases as n increases. Seagar *et al* (1987) derived the same result using a different approach where the best injection current is the one which maximizes the structural information about the object.

By solving Laplace's equation in polar coordinates using equation (12.4) as the Neumann boundary condition, the boundary voltage is expressed as

$$V_n(\theta) = C_n \cos n\theta + D_n \sin n\theta \quad (n = 1, 2, ...). \tag{12.5}$$

Assuming that $B_n = 0$, Seagar *et al* (1984, 1987) expressed the relationship between $J_n(\theta)$ and $V_n(\theta)$ as follows:

$$z_{nn} = \frac{V_n}{J_n} = \frac{C_n}{A_n} = -\frac{r_\mathrm{b}}{n\sigma_\mathrm{b}} \frac{(1+\alpha) + (1-\alpha)\beta^n}{(1+\alpha) - (1-\alpha)\beta^n} \tag{12.6}$$

and

$$\beta = \frac{r_\mathrm{a}^2}{r_\mathrm{b}^2} \tag{12.7}$$

where z_{nn} is the driving point impedance and α is the conductivity contrast defined earlier. When $\alpha = 1$ (i.e. homogeneous object), the driving point impedance is

$$z_{nn\mathrm{h}} = -\frac{r_\mathrm{b}}{n\sigma_\mathrm{b}} \tag{12.8}$$

and

$$V_{n\mathrm{h}} = z_{nn\mathrm{h}} J_n. \tag{12.9}$$

We can see that z_{nnh} does not contain any structural information.

12.2.2 Visibility

Seagar *et al* (1984) defined the visibility v_n as follows:

$$v_n = \frac{V_n - V_{nh}}{V_n + V_{nh}} = \frac{z_{nn} - z_{nnh}}{z_{nn} + z_{nnh}} \tag{12.10}$$

where V_n is the measured boundary voltage for the object with an anomaly at the center and V_{nh} is the boundary voltage for the homogeneous object. Substituting equation (12.6) and equation (12.8) into equation (12.10), we have

$$v_n = \frac{(1-\alpha)\beta^n}{1+\alpha}. \tag{12.11}$$

Figure 12.2 shows the visibility, v_1 and v_2, as a function of $\ln(\alpha)$ for several different values of β. For a given α, the anomaly is more visible for larger β (i.e. larger r_a). The smallest value of r_a for which the visibility is greater than the accuracy of the measurements is the limit to the size of the visible anomaly.

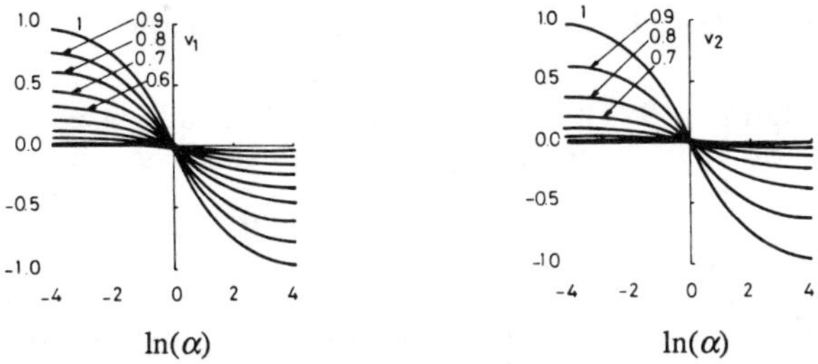

Figure 12.2 Visibility v_n for $n = 1$ and 2 as a function of $\ln(\alpha)$, with β as parameter (Seagar *et al* 1984).

12.2.3 Sensitivity

Sensitivity is defined as a fractional change in voltage for a fractional change in conductivity contrast. For cosine injection currents,

$$V_n(\theta) = A_n z_{nn} \cos n\theta. \tag{12.12}$$

By differentiating equation (12.12) with respect to α and multiplying by $\alpha/V_n(\theta)$, we have

$$s_n = \left[\frac{\delta V}{V} \Big/ \frac{\delta\alpha}{\alpha}\right]_n = \frac{-4\alpha\beta^n}{(1+\alpha)^2 - (1-\alpha)^2\beta^n} \tag{12.13}$$

where s_n is the sensitivity, $\delta V/V$ is the fractional change in voltage or the maximal admissible noise, and $\delta\alpha/\alpha$ is the conductivity resolution.

Figure 12.3 plots the sensitivity, s_1 and s_2, as a function of $\ln(\alpha)$ for several different values of β. For any given value of β, the sensitivity decreases as $|\ln(\alpha)|$ increases. The smallest change in α for which the sensitivity is greater than the accuracy of the measurements is the limit to the contrast of the anomaly.

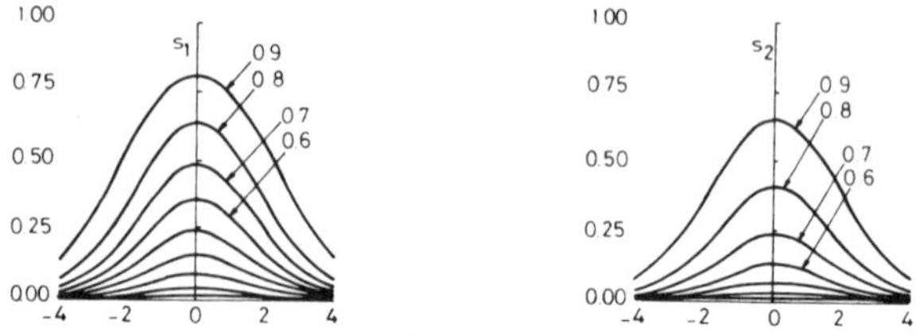

Figure 12.3 Sensitivity s_n for $n = 1$ and 2 as a function of $\ln(\alpha)$, with β as parameter (Seagar *et al* 1984).

12.2.4 Conformal transformation for an offset anomaly

Seagar and Bates (1985) and Seagar *et al* (1987) used a conformal transformation shown in figure 12.4 for the similar analysis using an object with an offset anomaly shown in figure 12.4(*b*).

Electrode position

Here we assume that we use two electrodes for current injection and discuss the best locations of the current injection electrodes. One of the factors in acquiring the maximal spatial resolution lies in forcing the current density distribution to be greatest in the region of interest. In order to maximize the measured voltage change for a change in tissue conductivity, the best electrode positions can be chosen which place the largest currents in the area of the anomaly.

From equations (12.11) and (12.13), we can find that the maximal visibility and sensitivity are achieved when $n = 1$ (fundamental spatial frequency of voltage and current density distribution). Therefore, the injection current should be the one which maximizes the fundamental spatial frequency component. The injection current chosen this way also maximizes the change in the boundary voltage between the objects with and without an anomaly. Note that this concept is equivalent to the definition of the distinguishability in Section 12.4. For a system with multiple current sources, we can achieve this by injecting $\cos(\theta)$.

For an object with an anomaly at the center as shown in figure 12.4(*a*), the best locations of the two current electrodes are at $\psi = \pm 90°$ (diagonal injection). For the object in figure 12.4(*b*), the best electrode locations can be determined by the conformal transformation and are shown in figure 12.5 as a function of the offset c for several different values of the radius ρ.

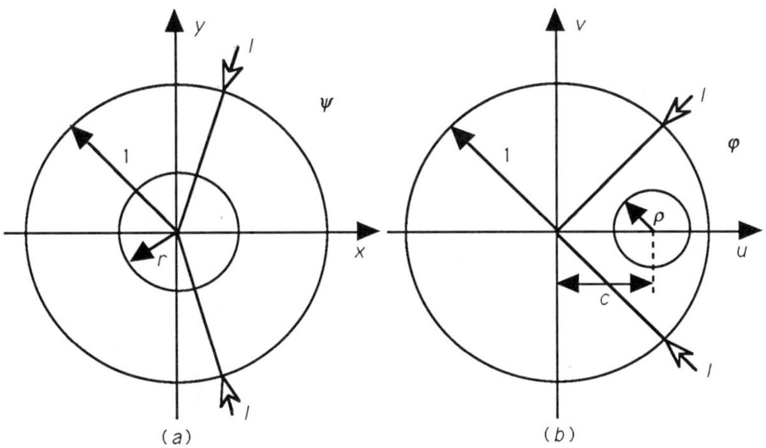

$$z = x + iy$$
$$z = (d - w)/(wd - 1)$$
$$r = [1 - c^2 + \rho^2 - \{(1 - c^2 + \rho^2)^2 - 4\rho^2\}^{1/2}]/2\rho$$
$$d = [1 + c^2 - \rho^2 - \{(1 + c^2 - \rho^2)^2 - 4\rho^2\}^{1/2}]/2c$$
$$\rho = r(1 - d^2)/(1 - r^2 d^2)$$
$$c = d(1 - r^2)/(1 - r^2 d^2)$$
$$w = u + iv$$
$$w = (d + z)/(d - z)$$

Figure 12.4 Conformal transformation between a circle of radius r at the center and a circle of radius ρ at the distance c from the origin. The unit circle is invariant under the transformation. I indicates the injection of current.

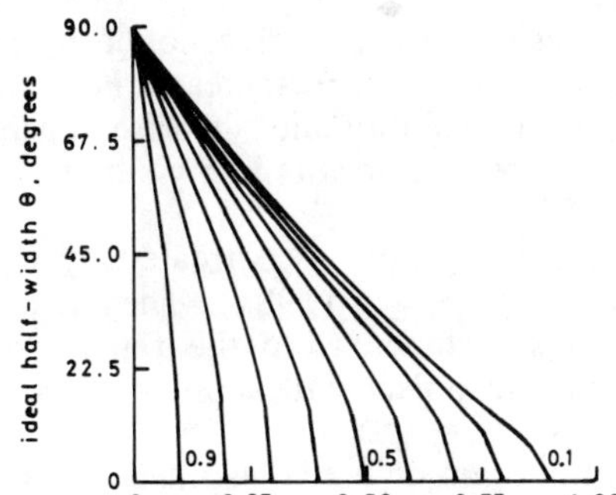

Figure 12.5 Best electrode positions for the object in figure 12.4(b). The curves are shown for the radius of the anomaly from 0.9 to 0.1 in steps of 0.1 (Seagar and Bates 1985).

Maximal visibility and sensitivity

From equations (12.11) and (12.13), the maximal magnitude of visibility and sensitivity are achieved when $n = 1$, $\alpha = 0$ or ∞ and $n = 1$, $\alpha = 1$, respectively. Also the maximal magnitudes are both equal to β which is r^2 for the object in figure 12.4(a). By using the conformal transformation shown in figure 12.4, figures 12.6(a) and (b) show the maximal visibility and sensitivity for the objects in figures 12.4(a) and (b), respectively. Each graph is plotted with the maximal sensitivity or visibility normalized to one along the y-axis.

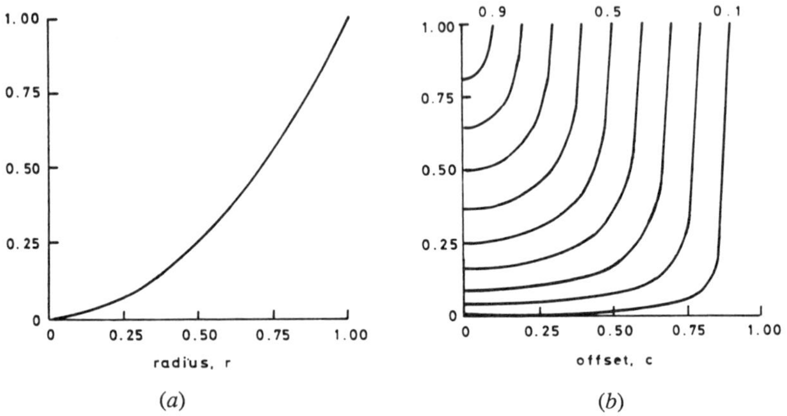

Figure 12.6 Maximal magnitude of visibility and sensitivity for (a) the object in figure 12.4(a) and (b) the object in figure 12.4(b). The curves in (b) are shown for the radius of the anomaly from 0.9 to 0.1 in steps of 0.1 (Seagar and Bates 1985).

Figure 12.6(a) shows that the visibility and sensitivity of centered objects increase by a factor of r^2. Figure 12.6(b) shows the offset object case where each line represents the radius of an anomaly with the smallest size beginning on the right. In figure 12.6(b), the visibility and sensitivity increase somewhat slowly as the offset increases until a certain threshold is reached where visibility increases rapidly with a very small offset increase. For example, an object of radius 0.1 will have almost no visibility until its offset reaches 0.75. However, an offset increase from 0.75 to 0.85 results in a visibility increase from 0.1 to 1.0, an increase of almost 90%.

Objects having flat geometry were also treated by a similar conformal transformation by Seagar and Bates (1985). They showed that visibility decreases as an anomaly's distance from the flat surface increases. The visibility and sensitivity of an object will approach zero as the depth of an anomaly increases.

In each case the visibility of an object is also dependent on its conductivity contrast with the surrounding medium. However, for given conductivity values the sensitivity can be known as a function of position as outlined here. For each geometry, we can use the maximal sensitivity to determine the best spatial resolution of an object in a given system. While each relationship is developed for one independent measurement, the actual spatial resolution can be improved for multiple measurements.

Practical experiments using two current sources and 32 voltage-measuring electrodes have shown visibilities as high as 0.62 (Seagar and Bates 1985). This value was obtained with the best electrode placement for an anomaly of radius 0.69 and offset of approximately 0.3. Figure 12.7 shows the plots of the maximal visibility measured experimentally for the objects in figures 12.4(*a*) and (*b*). The close agreement between the theoretical and measured values of visibility indicates the direct correlation between visibility and spatial resolution of an EIT system. They also discuss objects with different types of anomalies in circular geometry.

Note that the inherent visibility of an object can only be sensed if the errors in measurement are less than the voltage potential changes on the body periphery. Thus, the maximal visibility cannot be measured in absolute terms, but can only be measured in relation to the best possible image given the inherent errors of the tomography system. Therefore, an object which is readily visible in one system due to its contrast and position may be totally unrecognized in another system with larger measurement errors and a poorer reconstruction algorithm.

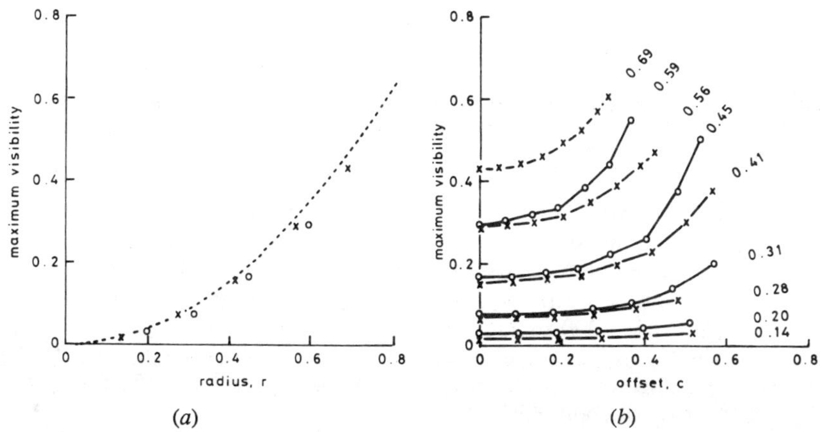

Figure 12.7 Maximal magnitude of visibility measured experimentally for (*a*) the object in figure 12.4(*a*) and (*b*) the object in figure 12.4(*b*). × and o indicate conducting and nonconducting anomalies, respectively. The dotted line in (*a*) shows the theoretical maximum. The curves in (*b*) are shown for the radius of the anomaly from 0.9 to 0.1 in steps of 0.1 (Seagar and Bates 1985).

12.3 RELATIONSHIPS AMONG SPATIAL RESOLUTION, CONDUCTIVITY RESOLUTION, CONTRAST AND NOISE

12.3.1 Relationships for an object with an anomaly at the center

Equation (12.13) not only defines the sensitivity but provides the relationships among spatial resolution $\beta^{1/2}$, noise $\delta V/V$, conductivity contrast α and conductivity resolution $\delta\alpha/\alpha$ for the object shown in figure 12.1(*a*) or figure 12.4(*a*). Figure 12.8 shows three plots indicating the relationships among sensitivity, spatial resolution, and conductivity contrast using the best single measurement with multiple current sources for a center anomaly.

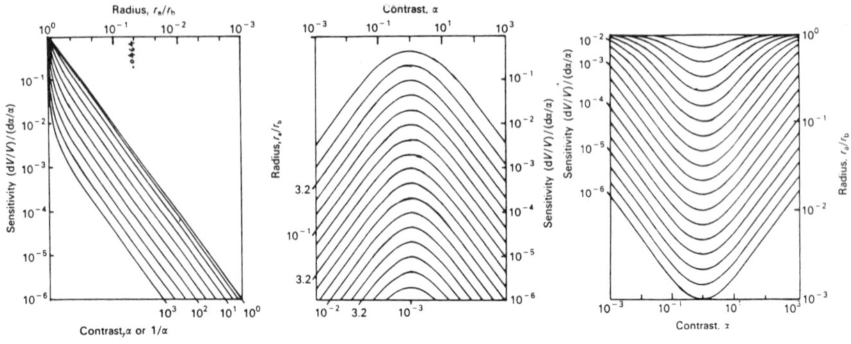

(*a*) (*b*) (*c*)

Figure 12.8 Relationship among sensitivity, spatial resolution and conductivity contrast for (*a*) particular values of contrast, (*b*) particular values of radius and (*c*) particular values of sensitivity (Seagar *et al* 1987).

As an example, what is the accuracy of a tomography system which has a noise ratio of one part in 10^5 ($\delta V/V = 10^{-5}$), a spatial resolution of 1 in 10 ($r_a/r_b = 0.1$), and a conductivity in a contrast range of 1000 to 1? On figure 12.8(*a*), find the radius ratio of 0.1 or 10^{-1} at the top. Move vertically down until the contrast is 1000 to 1 or the 10^3 line is intersected, a line is drawn horizontally to the point on the sensitivity scale where the number 3×10^{-5} is approximated. The conductivity resolution is then given by $10^{-5}/(3 \times 10^{-5}) = 0.3$ or an accuracy of about 30%.

Based on the plots in figure 12.8, the relationships can be summarized as follows (Seagar *et al* 1987):

(1) degrading $\delta\alpha/\alpha$ by K balances improving $\beta^{1/2}$ by $K^{1/2}$
(2) improving $\delta V/V$ by K balances improving $\beta^{1/2}$ by $K^{1/2}$
(3) improving $\delta V/V$ by K balances improving $\delta\alpha/\alpha$ by K
(4) extending α by K balances degrading $\beta^{1/2}$ by $K^{1/2}$
(5) extending α by K balances degrading $\delta\alpha/\alpha$ by K
(6) extending α by K balances improving $\delta V/V$ by K

These results show that the spatial resolution is least sensitive to changes in the other variables. For example, an improvement in noise by a factor of 10 could produce an improvement in the conductivity resolution by the same factor but in the spatial resolution only by a factor of $10^{1/2}$ (≈ 3.2). Also, note that we need an improvement in noise by 1000 to obtain an improvement both in conductivity resolution and spatial resolution by 10. These plots can also be used to determine the value of one parameter when the others are known.

Use of multiple independent measurements might be able to improve the spatial and conductivity resolution. However, Seagar *et al* (1987) argued that for a small anomaly (radius of 0.4 or less), more than one independent measurement does not significantly improve the conductivity resolution (accuracy) further based on their error analysis.

12.3.2 Relationships for an object with an offset anomaly

The conformal transformation shown in figure 12.4 provides the relationship among c, ρ and r shown in figure 12.9. Using the two plots in figure 12.9, in symmetric geometry we can find the value of r which corresponds to the values of c and ρ in offset geometry. Therefore, the results in the previous section can be applied to the object with an offset anomaly shown in figure 12.4(b) after the conformal transformation.

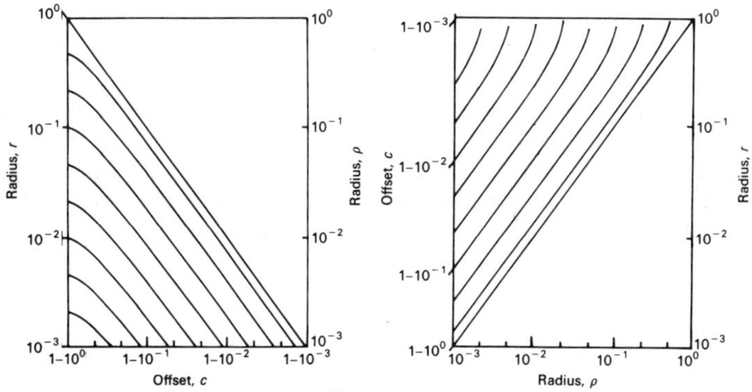

(a) (b)

Figure 12.9 Relationships among r, c and ρ. (Seagar *et al* 1987).

12.3.3 Spatial resolution

In figure 12.1(b) and figure 12.4(b), the way in which the spatial resolution varies is dependent on the object's position c from the center of the object, its radius r_a (or ρ) and its conductivity σ_a. Additionally, for a system with two current sources, the object's visibility will increase as the position of a current-injecting electrode approaches ϕ in figure 12.1(b).

In figure 12.9(a), for any fixed value of r, the radius ρ decreases as the offset c increases. Therefore, at the object's center, the spatial resolution will be poorest, becoming better as it approaches the surface. With the body radius normalized to one, the spatial resolution of the offset object will vary according to the relationship $1/(1 - c^2)$ (Seagar *et al* 1987). Note that this relationship holds only when other parameters of the system are held constant, i.e., an anomaly near the body surface surrounded by tissue of similar conductivity may in fact have poorer spatial resolution than centered objects with high contrast to the surrounding medium. Spatial resolution improves with the conductivity contrast of the region, the improved geometry used and the number of measurements taken.

By using the results in Section 12.3.1, we can generate the following table which shows the changes in the spatial resolution, conductivity resolution, visibility and sensitivity for variations in the offset c.

Table 12.1 Changes in the spatial resolution, conductivity resolution, visibility, and sensitivity for variations in the offset c.

Spatial resolution	$\frac{1}{1-c^2}$
Conductivity resolution	$\frac{1}{(1-c^2)^2}$
Visibility	$\frac{1}{(1-c^2)^2}$
Sensitivity	$\frac{1}{(1-c^2)^2}$

In multielectrode systems, the spatial resolution does nevertheless increase for voltage-sensing electrodes near current-injecting electrodes, where the gradient of the electric field is greatest. However, to determine overall spatial resolution we must consider other factors such as number of electrodes used, placement, method of current injection and reconstruction algorithms. Various parameters are here abstracted to illustrate the effects on resolution by changing one parameter at a time.

12.3.4 Conductivity contrast

In EIT, contrast in conductivity has a limited effect on changes in electrical potential measured at the electrodes. For example, while the conductivity changes associated with lung ventilation may range up to 100%, the corresponding changes in electrode potentials are typically 5% (Brown and Seagar 1987). Such small measured voltage changes provide an absolute limit on the ability for imaging conductivities that vary little from their surrounding media. ADCs have a quantization error for a 12 bit system of $1/2^{12}$. In practice, tissue conductivity changes of 3% relative to surrounding tissue require the voltage profile on the periphery to have an accuracy of 0.1%, an accuracy which is extremely difficult to achieve given that electrode spacings need to have a similar accuracy (see Section 9.3). However, dynamic imaging eliminates some of the largest measurement errors (i.e., precise knowledge of electrode spacing), and sensitivity to changes in voltage profiles of 0.1% are possible (Seagar *et al* 1987).

The effect of conductivity contrast on image visibility is dependent on spatial resolution. The visibility and sensitivity of an object with a given conductivity contrast decreases with its depth in the medium. From equations (12.11) and (12.13), letting the conductivity contrast α be equal to 0.4 with a spatial resolution $\beta^{1/2}$ of 0.2 will give a visibility of 0.025 and a sensitivity of 0.033. Both sensitivity and visibility are increased significantly by holding α constant and increasing the spatial resolution $\beta^{1/2}$ to 0.9. This gives a visibility of 0.27 and a sensitivity of 0.78.

In situations where the conductivity of an object varies little from its surrounding region, multiple independent measurements may be needed to improve visibility. Consider a situation where conductivity contrast is such that the corresponding changes in peripheral voltage measurements compare with the level of measurement error within the system. Under these conditions, the object will not be visible when only a single measurement is used. As the number of independent measurements is increased, the relative error decreases for objects to be visible.

12.3.5 Conductivity resolution and multiple anomalies

Conductivity resolution was defined as the smallest difference of conductivity of a region that can be detected. Letting the conductivity contrast be α, the conductivity resolution was determined algebraically as $\delta\alpha/\alpha$, the percent change in conductivity contrast. The accuracy is equal to the conductivity resolution. This resolution significantly affects the degree of sensitivity of voltage measurement, i.e., the departure in $V(\theta)$ from its value for a homogeneous region. Sensitivity was defined as a fractional change in voltage for a fractional change in contrast (conductivity resolution) in equation (12.13).

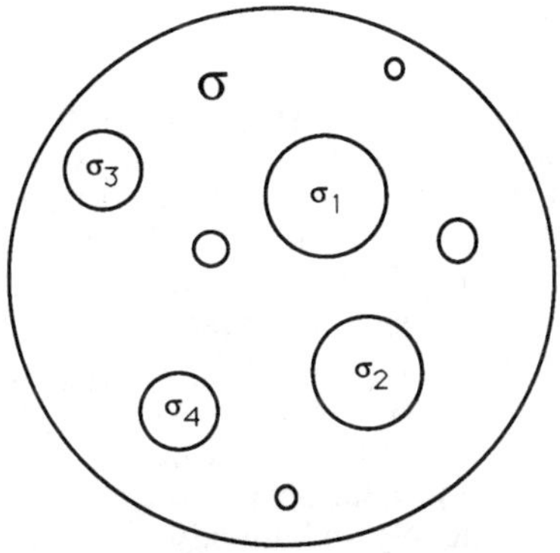

Figure 12.10 Conductivity model for multiple offset anomalies.

In many practical situations of impedance imaging, in an inhomogeneous region multiple anomalies exist which obscure the conductivity contrast of the region of interest. Figure 12.10 models multiple anomalies within a homogeneous medium. The degree of interference between interior anomalies is a function of the distances from the body surface, their relative distances from each other, their relative sizes and their relative conductivity contrasts with the surrounding medium. Under certain conditions, however, it is possible to ignore their interrelationships and treat the contribution to the surface potential of each object as being independent of all other interior anomalies. This occurs when neighboring anomalies are sufficiently small and deep within the body so as to be negligible. In practice, the degree to which multiple interior anomalies are invisible for these reasons corresponds directly to image quality for a single anomaly in the presence of surrounding anomalies.

Seagar and Bates (1985) calculated the relative conductivity interference for five discrete anomalies in the human calf. Figure 12.11 shows the model for this conductivity. The conductivity of the surrounding medium was normalized to

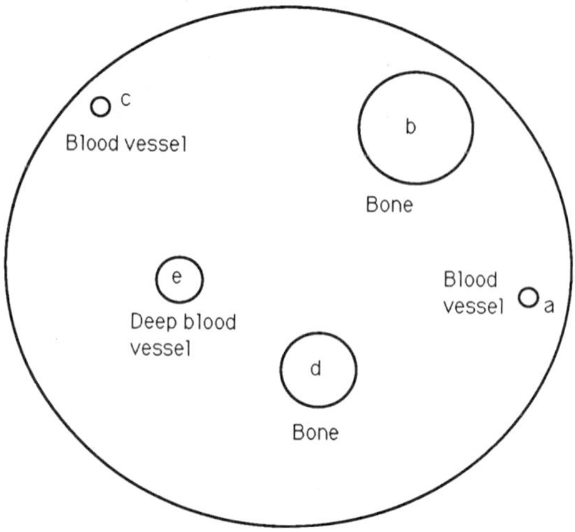

Figure 12.11 Conductivity cross section of the human leg at calf level.

unity with two bones and three blood vessels of infinite and zero conductivity, respectively. Anomalies of high conductivity contrast with respect to a homogeneous medium, i.e., the bones labeled (b) and (d), have visibilities which dominate the effects of interference due to coupling. Coupling is also less of a factor in bone (b) which is closer to the periphery and exhibits more conductivity resolution than the smaller bone (d) in figure 12.11.

When attempting to image a single anomaly in the presence of multiple offset anomalies, it is sometimes convenient to invoke *a priori* knowledge of the conductivity distribution within the reconstruction algorithm. Accounting for multiple offsets in the backprojection technique, it is possible to image a specific region of interest uniquely and directly.

12.4 DISTINGUISHABILITY

Seagar *et al* (1984) and Seagar and Bates (1985) defined the visibility as a measure of the ability to qualitatively distinguish between different conductivities. In contrast, distinguishability is the measure of the ability of a pattern of currents to distinguish between two conductivities. To determine distinguishability, let the measured voltage at a point p be $V(p)$. Then,

$$V(p) = [R(\sigma)j](p) \tag{12.14}$$

where $R(\sigma)$ is a linear operator, which depends nonlinearly on the conductivity σ, and j is the injection current.

In figure 12.12, we wish to distinguish between the unknown medium σ_1 (which has an object in the center with conductivity ω) and the conjectured medium σ_0 (which has no object). These media are distinguishable if

$$\delta = \delta(j) = \frac{\|R(\sigma_1)j - R(\sigma_0)j\|}{\|j\|} > \varepsilon \tag{12.15}$$

where δ is the distinguishability, ε is the measurement precision (for example in a 12 bit system, $1/2^{12}$), and $\|\ \|$ is the norm.

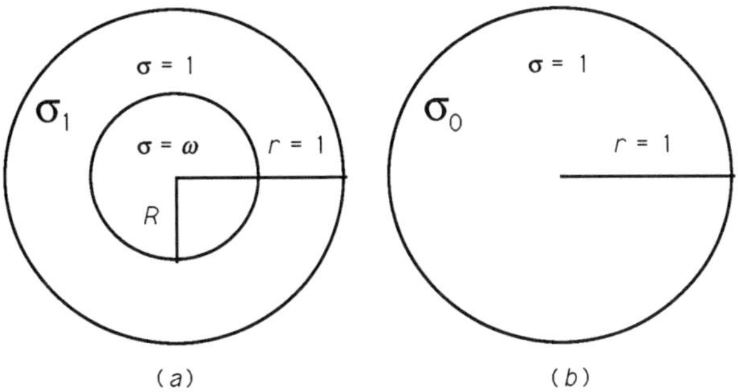

Figure 12.12 Distinguishability is the measure of the magnitude of voltage difference between (*a*) unknown nonhomogeneous medium σ_1 and (*b*) conjectured homogeneous medium σ_0 normalized.

Isaacson (1986) and Gisser *et al* (1987) developed methods for maximizing distinguishability for cylindrical geometries and also for arbitrary geometries. The currents that maximize distinguishability are called the optimal currents. The optimal currents for distinguishing between an arbitrary σ_1 and σ_0 are found through an iterative process called the power method and deflation technique.

Since σ's in the body are unknown, they cannot be determined without experiment. In maximizing distinguishability, an interactive experimental process must be pursued to approximate the best current j_b to distinguish between σ_1 and σ_0. These steps involve guessing a injection current density $j_k(\theta)$ $(k = 0)$ and measuring the resulting voltage when applying $j_k(\theta)$ to the bodies of conductivity σ_1 and σ_0. The normalized difference between these two voltages gives the next injection current $j_{k+1}(\theta)$. The magnitude of the current difference between j_{k+1} and j_k is then compared with the measurement precision error ε. The iteration index k is then incremented until the measurement precision is reached.

For the special case of a circular disk, the optimal currents for a given number of electrodes n are applied at angles governed by the trigonometric function

$$j_n(\theta) = \cos n(\theta - \theta_0)/\pi^{1/2} \quad \text{for any } \theta_0 \tag{12.16}$$

where $n = 1, 2, \ldots, N$ and N is the total number of injection currents. This yields a distinguishability of

$$\delta_n = 2\,|\mu|\,\alpha_n \tag{12.17}$$

where $\alpha_n = r^{2n}/[n(1 + \mu r^{2n})]$ and $\mu = (\omega - 1)/(\omega + 1)$.

The practical usefulness of the concept of distinguishability is that it provides a way of determining optimal patterns of injection currents which maximize the distinguishability or visibility for an arbitrary conductivity distribution. A further discussion about this iterative procedure is described in Section 8.6.

12.5 TEMPORAL RESOLUTION

The most investigated areas in dynamically resolving body resistivity changes have been in the areas of respiratory investigations, cardiac-related changes and monitoring of gastric emptying.

Gastric emptying can be monitored because acid secretion or the emptying of a meal from the stomach will alter the distribution of conductivity in the upper abdomen. Mangnall *et al* (1987) conducted experiments on 19 subjects whereby 16 electrodes were evenly placed in an array around the upper abdomen. For the 16-electrode array, 208 measurements were made during each cycle lasting about 100 ms. Data sets were then backprojected with an initial data set to form a cross-sectional image.

Ventilation can be monitored due to variations in conductivity between inspiration and expiration. The magnitude of the conductivity changes varies according to the size and shape of the patient thus making quantitative measurements of volume difficult. However, EIT can be used in monitoring the rate and depth of ventilation as well as in detecting pulmonary edema where fluid increase in the lungs causes a change in conductivity. Long-term monitoring of ventilation can be achieved by averaging several hundred data collection cycles over a period of a few minutes.

Cardiac-related changes can be monitored due to conductivity changes when blood is ejected and replaced by ventricular muscle. Also, changes in the major arteries will take place as vessels expand and contract with blood. These changes are the ones which are used in determining cardiac output. Changes of blood vessel diameter of 1% can be seen by gated cardiac imaging averaged over 50 cardiac cycles with images collected at intervals of 100 ms (Brown *et al* 1987).

Dynamic imaging allows very sensitive impedance measurements to be made whereby resistivity changes as low as 1% can be seen. In dynamic imaging, the backprojection of a collected data set against an initial data set can be used to avoid the need for electrode positions to be precisely known. For example, a 2% fall in lung tissue resistivity or a change of blood vessel diameter by 1% during systole can be seen in the imaging process. However, movement artifact levels are often higher in moving body tissues requiring signal averaging to give adequate SNR in the images. For cardiac cycle imaging, as many as 50 data sets synchronized to the ECG may need to be collected to minimize interference from movement artifacts.

A major drawback in EIT is the relatively poor spatial resolution. Increasing the number of electrodes allows more independent measurements to be made. Subsequently, greater spatial resolution can be achieved within a limit. However, this results in an increase in data collection time which degrades the SNR. For dynamic imaging, data collection time must be kept low to avoid blurring due to changing resistivity distributions. Spatial resolutions of approximately 10% have been obtained by Eyuboglu *et al* (1987), for cardiac activity. This low spatial resolution prevents distinguishing of the heart chambers and blood vessels. Figure 12.13 shows several regions which were distinguishable in dynamic imaging of the thorax. The impedance variations were then compared with an electrocardiogram and proved to be synchronous, although some organs were difficult to define clearly due to low spatial resolution.

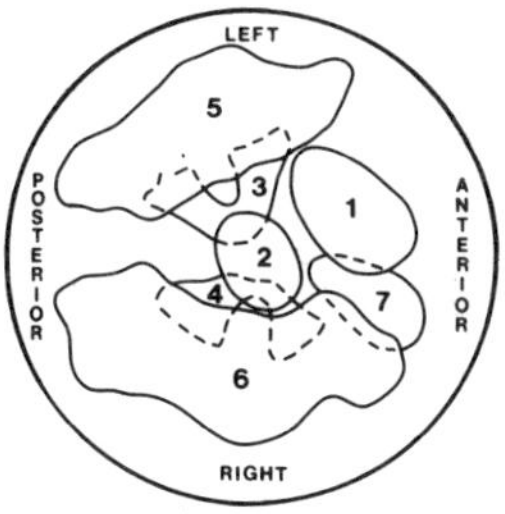

Figure 12.13 The seven regions which can be recognized in the ECG-gated images of the thorax. These regions correspond to: 1 ventricles, 2 aorta, 3 and 4 pulmonary arteries, 5 and 6 left and right lungs, 7 right atria and vena cavae. Due to the low resolution of the system, it is difficult to separate some of the organs such as the heart chambers and especially the vena cavae and right atrium (Eyuboglu *et al* 1987).

12.6 DISCUSSION

Note that the performance is related to the purpose for which the imaging system is used. In some cases amplitude accuracy is not as important as the mere ability to detect a difference in body conductivity in a certain region. We must make various trade-offs between visibility, sensitivity, spatial resolution, conductivity contrast, conductivity resolution (accuracy) and SNR to develop the optimal system for resolving objects of different conductivity, size and location in the body.

12.7 STUDY QUESTIONS

12.1. Define spatial resolution and give the best spatial resolution that has been achieved in a physical phantom.

12.2. Define conductivity resolution and give the best conductivity resolution that has been obtained in a physical phantom.

12.3. Define conductivity contrast and give the best conductivity contrast that has been obtained in a physical phantom.

12.4 Define visibility and sensitivity.

12.5 What is the accuracy of an EIT system which has a noise ratio of one part in 10^4 ($\delta V/V = 10^{-4}$), a spatial resolution of 1 in 10 ($r_a/r_b = 0.1$) and a conductivity contrast range of 500 to 1?

12.6 In figure 12.4(*b*), $c = 0.5$ and $\rho = 0.2$. Find the optimal electrode position (angle φ).
12.7 In figure 12.4(*b*), everything is fixed except c. Plot spatial resolution and conductivity resolution as a function of c.
12.8 Describe the relationship between visibility and spatial resolution.
12.9 You have a 12 bit EIT system with a measurement precision of 1/4096. You decided to improve the spatial resolution of the system by a factor of 10. What is the required measurement precision of the new EIT system and how many bits do you need?
12.10 Define distinguishability and give the best distinguishability that has been achieved in a physical phantom.
12.11 Compare visibility with distinguishability.
12.12 You have an EIT system with 32 independent current sources and 32 electrodes. Describe the procedure of finding the optimal patterns of injection current which provide the maximal distinguishability.
12.13 Define temporal resolution and give the best temporal resolution that has been obtained in a physical phantom.
12.14 You decided to develop an EIT system with 32 electrodes to study cardiac-related changes and to monitor ventilation. Find the required temporal resolution in both cases.
12.15 Give equations that relate as many of the above variables as possible.

13

Clinical Applications

Sudhakar Bhat

Electrical Impedance Tomography (EIT) can be used in a wide range of clinical applications, at a low cost and without any known hazard. The biological tissues have a wide range of resistivities (figure 2.13). This implies that we can obtain good tissue contrast in EIT imaging.

This chapter describes the various applications in the medical field, some of which have been demonstrated and some of which are speculations. To date, very few *in vivo* measurements have been obtained, which are described in the sections to follow. EIT can produce both static and dynamic images (Section 1.5). The electrical impedance approach is a noninvasive method, and hence should be useful for clinical assessment of patients.

13.1 CARDIAC PARAMETERS

Most presently used methods for the measurement of cardiac parameters (Cardiac Output, CO; Stroke Volume, SV; and Left Ventricular Ejection Time, LVET) are invasive, and require cardiac or arterial catheterization. This has restricted their wide application. The invasive techniques include CO measurement by the Direct Fick principle, dye-dilution method, thermodilution method and many others. The Direct Fick principle and the dye-dilution method require the withdrawal of blood, thereby restricting the number of readings that can be taken (Porter and Swain 1987).

Atzler and Lehmann in 1932 found that the changes in transthoracic impedance could be related to the events in the cardiac cycle. Kubicek *et al* (1974) using this principle developed an impedance plethysmograph called the Minnesota Impedance Cardiograph (MIC), which can be used to measure the CO, SV and the contractility of the heart. They used four aluminized Mylar strip electrodes. Measurement of CO is made by placing two electrodes around the neck, and two around the abdomen. A constant sinusoidal AC current of 4 mA RMS at 100 kHz is passed between the outer two electrodes (1 and 4), and the changes in thoracic impedance are calculated by measuring the voltage between the inner two electrodes (2 and 3). We can then calculate the ventricular stroke volume in liters,

$$\mathrm{SV} = \rho \left(\frac{L}{Z_0}\right)^2 T \left(\frac{dZ}{dt}\right)_{\min} \tag{13.1}$$

where ρ = resistivity of blood (at 100 kHz) ≅ 1.45 ±2% Ω m (at 37.5°C), L = mean distance between the inner electrodes (2 and 3), in meters, Z_0 = mean thoracic impedance between electrodes (2 and 3), in ohms, T = left ventricular ejection time (obtained from the dZ/dt waveform), in seconds, and $(dZ/dt)_{\min}$ = minimum value of (dZ/dt) occurring during the cardiac cycle in ohms per second. Using the SV obtained from equation (13.1), and the heart rate (HR), we can calculate,

$$\mathrm{CO} = \mathrm{SV}\cdot\mathrm{HR} \quad \text{(liters/min)}. \tag{13.2}$$

EIT can be used to measure cardiac parameters noninvasively. Eyuboglu *et al* (1987) concluded that the thoracic impedance changes can be related to the cardiac cycle and hence can be inferred from the EIT images. They have shown, from the ECG-gated dynamic EIT images of the thorax (figure 12.13), that the change in the thoracic impedance (related to the cardiac activity) from different organs can be distinguished. They used 16 Ag–AgCl ECG electrodes, all equally spaced, and placed around the chest at the nipple level. A current of 5 mA (peak-to-peak) at 50 kHz is applied between any two adjacent electrodes, and voltages measured between all other adjacent pairs of electrodes. This process is repeated for all pairs of current electrodes. The Sheffield system (Brown and Seagar 1987) makes the $104 = [E(E-1)/2]$ independent measurements in 41.6 ms, thereby giving 24 frames of data each second (= 1000/41.6).

In order to reduce the noise level and the effect due to respiratory changes, they used an ECG R-wave trigger and collected 30 frames from the thorax. They then averaged the data from 100 cardiac cycles. This improved the SNR by a factor of 10 (Newman 1978). The Sheffield group obtained dynamic images of the cardiac cycle, which showed the resistivity changes within the thorax. Blood has a lower impedance than the other tissues of chest. Cardiac systole is characterized by ventricular contraction with blood flowing continuously to the periphery due to the distension of the aorta, and is therefore, accompanied by an increase in impedance across the chest. Diastole, which is characterized by the ventricular relaxation with blood perfusing in, leads to a decrease in impedance. Figures 13.1(*a*) and (*b*) show the electrode positions around the body.

Though the Sheffield group has not obtained high-resolution images, it seems likely that we could make use of the high speed and sensitivity to measure the cardiac parameters. The profile of the impedance change, which is used to reconstruct the image, can be used to calculate these parameters. Figure 13.2 shows 13 of the 104 profiles of the impedance change waveforms at peak systole obtained by the Sheffield group, which were used to reconstruct the image. The blood, having a high conductivity, gives rise to an appreciable change in impedance during cardiac systole. Therefore, the biggest change in impedance could be related to the heart (in figure 13.2, it would be the fifth waveform from the top). We speculate that this change in impedance waveform could be used to calculate the stroke volume (SV) and the cardiac output (CO). Equation (13.1) could be used to obtain SV, once the first derivative (dZ/dt) is obtained from the impedance waveform (the baseline impedance, Z_0, can also

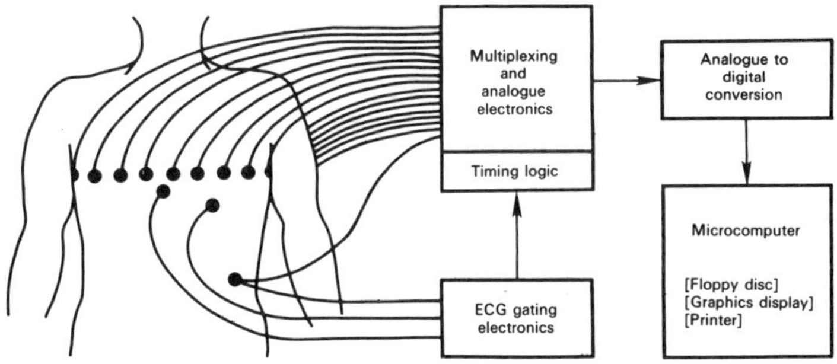

(*a*)

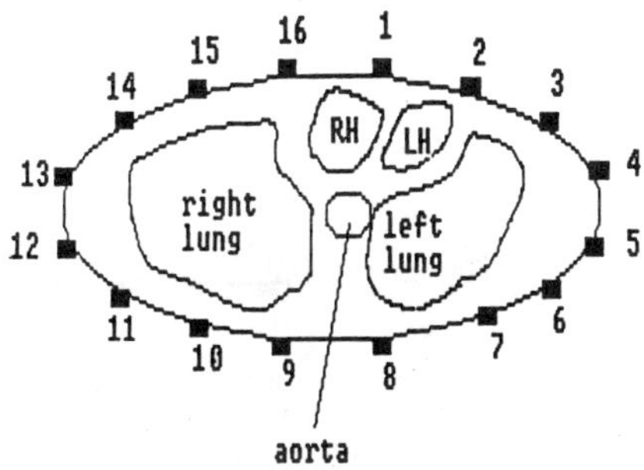

(*b*)

Figure 13.1 (*a*) Electrodes are placed on the chest at the nipple level for the ECG-gated EIT imaging system. (*b*) Cross-sectional view of the chest showing different regions and the electrode positions (Brown *et al* 1987).

be obtained from the same waveform). Another way would be to record (dZ/dt), and then use that information to obtain the SV from equation (13.1), and hence the CO.

Eyuboglu *et al* (1989) have measured the position-dependent point response function (PRF) for the Sheffield system to find the limitations of stroke volume determination using impedance imaging. They found that object sensitivity decreases from periphery to center and also with distance from the plane of the electrodes in three dimensions. Due to the highly position-dependent PRF of the EIT system, an accurate calculation of an index of cardiac volumes is complicated and calibration is needed.

13.2 CEREBRAL HEMODYNAMICS

The incidence of periventricular intraventricular hemorrhage in low birthweight infants (1500 g), or infants born after less than 35 weeks of gestation, is about 40 to 45% (Volpe 1981). This is a major cause of death in these infants.

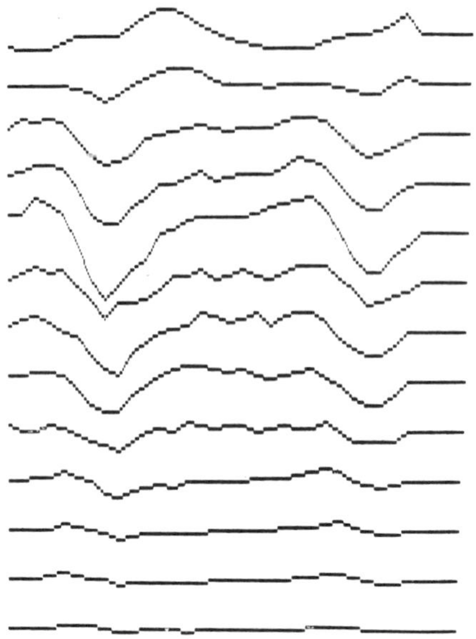

Figure 13.2 Thirteen of the 104 impedance profiles used to reconstruct an image during cardiac systole. The fifth waveform from the top has the maximal change in impedance, and hence could be related to the heart. This waveform could be used to obtain various cardiac parameters (Brown *et al* 1987).

Therefore, early detection of the intraventricular hemorrhage (IVH) in these infants would be useful.

The most reliable and convenient screening procedure is ultrasonic scanning, which uses a piezoelectric transducer applied to the skin over the anterior fontanelle. Ultrasonic scanning is usually done once in 24 h on a patient. Therefore, it becomes difficult to determine the exact time the hemorrhage occurred. If we could determine this, we could obtain a better insight into the etiology of IVH, which is not properly understood. Moreover, the infants in the risk group should be monitored closely, and kept under a constant watch.

Cerebrospinal fluid (CSF) is about 2-1/2 times as conductive as blood (see figure 2.13). IVH occurs when the fragile network of capillaries situated below the cerebral ventricles rupture, which leads to the oozing out of blood and mixing with the CSF in the ventricles, thereby increasing the impedance. This leads to the conclusion that impedance imaging in this case could be helpful.

Tarassenko *et al* (1985) used the principle of EIT to image the distribution of electrical resistivity in the brain. They placed 16 EEG electrodes on the infant's head, around the occipitofrontal circumference (OFC), passed a high-frequency ($\cong$ 50 kHz) 750 μA RMS current between a pair of opposite electrodes, and measured voltages between all other adjacent electrodes. They used the equipotential method to reconstruct the distribution of resistivity within the head. They first assumed a uniform resistivity, ρ_u, and then computed the peripheral potential, ΔV. Then they measured the potential, $\Delta V'$. They repeated this procedure for all sets of measurements. This yielded the new modified resistivity,

$$\rho_{\mathrm{n}} = \rho_{\mathrm{u}}\left(\frac{\Delta V'}{\Delta V}\right). \tag{13.3}$$

It takes a processing time of about 1/20th of a second. This gives a static image, by backprojecting the ratio ($\Delta V'/\Delta V$).

In particular, for IVH, we can use a dynamic image, for which we need not know the exact position of the electrodes. Here, we measure the peripheral voltages, before and after the hemorrhage occurs, at times t_1 and t_2. The two images obtained from these data are then subtracted to get an image of the change in resistivity between t_1 and t_2. Thus, in this case, equation (13.3) becomes

$$\rho_{\mathrm{n}} = \rho_{\mathrm{u}}\left(\frac{\Delta V'_{t_2} - \Delta V'_{t_1}}{\Delta V}\right). \tag{13.4}$$

Figure 13.3 shows a dynamic image reconstructed using a reference (initial) and another later set of data (Murphy *et al* 1987). The regions of high and low resistivities can be easily distinguished. Movement artifact seems to be a major problem in imaging the newborn. Murphy *et al* (1987) describe an effective algorithm to reject these corrupted data. The use of a low-pass filter would smooth the data, but increase the total frame acquisition time.

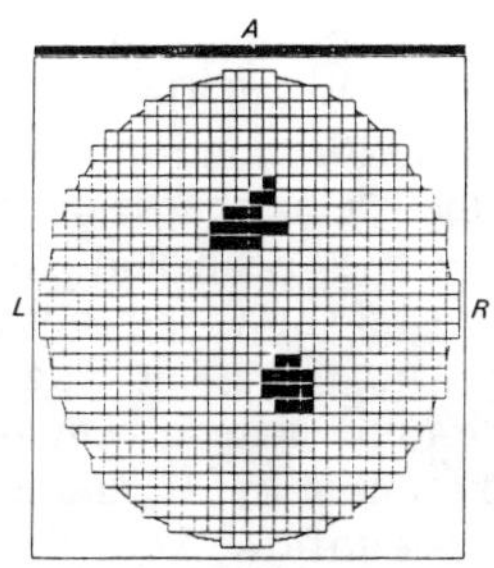

Figure 13.3 Image of the brain of a newborn, suffering from a major right-sided intraparenchymal hemorrhage. The dark regions show the increased resistivity due to the pooling-in of blood into the ventricles (Murphy *et al* 1987).

Static imaging could be very useful for the detection of IVH. But, prior to the backprojection, the knowledge of the exact position of the electrodes on the scalp would need to be determined in order to calculate the equipotential lines, and hence the reference set of voltage values. Moreover, the shape of the head varies to a great extent in the low-birthweight infants, and therefore, it would be extremely difficult to generate three-dimensional models of sufficient accuracy for good image reconstruction. It is therefore advisable to revert to the dynamic imaging technique, described above.

Tarassenko *et al* (1985) showed that impedance imaging improves as the resistivity ratio increases from 1 to 50. Higher resistivity ratios yield very little improvement over a ratio of 50 (figure 13.4).

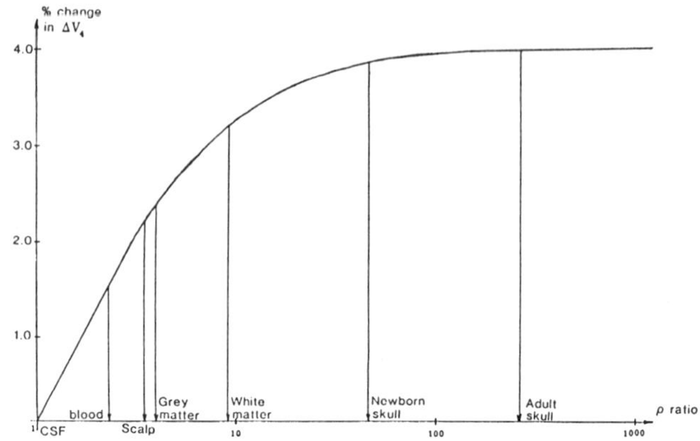

Figure 13.4 Percent change in peripheral potential measurement when the resistivity of a test region is increased (Tarassenko *et al* 1985).

13.3 LIMB PLETHYSMOGRAPHY

The measurement of peripheral blood flow is useful for the diagnosis of cardiovascular diseases, and also for monitoring vascular hemodynamics in the limb segments of patients in the ICU and those undergoing operations. The only accurate method available is venous occlusion plethysmography, but it is very cumbersome to apply. Figure 13.5 shows the sequence of operations in venous occlusion plethysmography. As the name suggests, the venous blood is prevented from leaving the limb by using a venous occlusion cuff. The limb is pressurized to 50 mm Hg. The initial linear, and then the exponential nature of the curve is due to the arterial inflow, which is defined as the increase in volume of blood in the limb per unit time. When the cuff is removed, the volume returns back to normal (figure 13.5, curve A). Curve B in figure 13.5 shows the slow return of volume, when a venous thrombosis partially blocks the return of venous blood (Webster 1978b).

Blood is among the most conductive fluids in the human body. Nyboer *et al* (1950) and many others showed that with the flow of blood into any segment of the limb, the volume of blood in that segment fluctuates, and hence, gives rise to an impedance decrease. Impedance also decreases with an increase in velocity of the blood (Liebman 1970). This fact has been corroborated by a number of researchers who made *in vitro* measurements of the impedance of blood under static and dynamic conditions.

In electrical impedance plethysmography, measurements are made by placing four circumferential electrodes around the body segment. A high-frequency

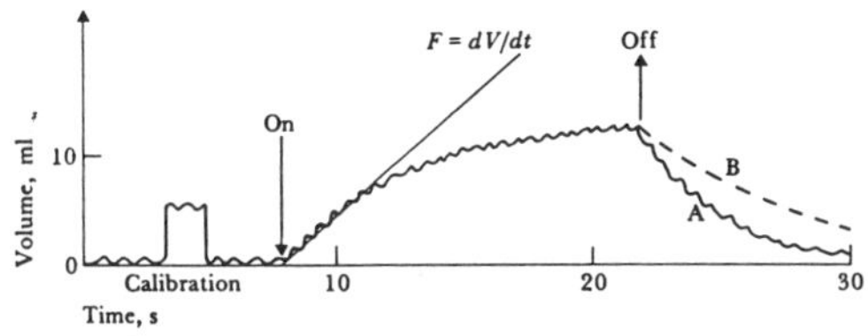

Figure 13.5 Principle of venous occlusion plethysmography (see text for details) (Webster 1978b).

(~ 100 kHz) AC current of 4 mA is passed between the two outer electrodes and the voltage measured between the inner ones. Impedance change permits calculation of the volume change in the body segment (Webster 1978b):

$$\Delta V = -\frac{\rho L^2 \Delta Z}{Z_0^2} \quad (\mathrm{m}^3) \tag{13.5}$$

where the symbols have their usual meaning (Section 13.1).

Kubicek showed that the above equation (13.5) can be put in an alternative form, in which we do not need to know the resistivity of blood:

$$\Delta V = \frac{C^2 L \Delta Z}{4\pi Z_0} \quad (\mathrm{m}^3) \tag{13.6}$$

where C is the circumference of the limb (m).

The limb blood flow is given by

$$\mathrm{LBF} = 60\frac{\Delta V}{\Delta t} \quad (\mathrm{m}^3/\mathrm{min}). \tag{13.7}$$

Cardiovascular disease leads to a reduction in blood flow to the extremities. Therefore, to assist in the diagnosis of peripheral vascular diseases, we need to measure the peripheral blood flow.

EIT could be used to measure the volume change of blood in the limb segment, and hence, the blood flow. EIT could also be used to detect blood clots (thrombi) in the deep veins of the leg, which is called deep venous thrombosis (DVT) (Luedtke *et al* 1987). In such a case, the blood circulation is hindered. The present techniques to detect DVT include venography, impedance plethysmography and doppler ultrasonography. Luedtke *et al* (1987) could reconstruct cross-sectional images using EIT. They placed 16 Ag/AgCl ECG electrodes circumferentially on the calf, as shown in figure 13.6. They applied a sinusoidal current at 50 kHz between the chosen current pair of electrodes and measured the differential voltages between the remaining electrode pairs. They first obtained an initial set of data with the subject lying down, and the leg raised to force the blood toward the heart, thereby causing the vein to collapse. As the blood moved out, a high-impedance region was created. The thigh was then pressurized to 50 mm Hg for about 5 min using a cuff, with the subject in a sitting position. This blocked the venous return flow, but allowed arterial blood to flow into the lower leg, thereby creating a low-impedance region. Thus, they obtained dynamic images. Figure 13.7 shows the reconstructed image. The bright spot located near the center of the calf is a low-impedance region. Note that they have not duplicated figure 13.5. In other words, using EIT, we cannot obtain as much quantitative information as when using venous occlusion plethysmography.

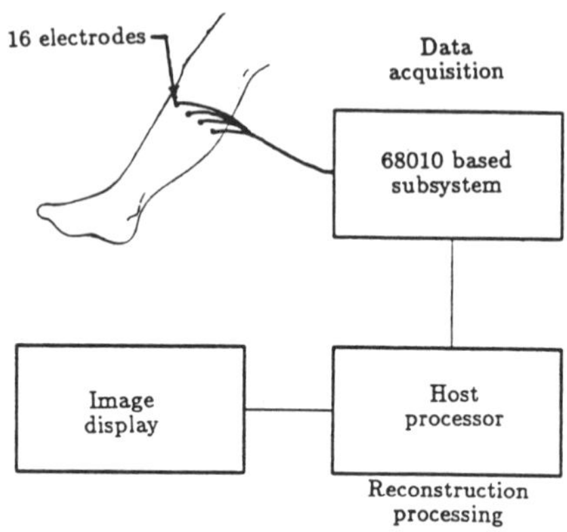

Figure 13.6 The electrode placement system for the detection of DVT in the human calf (Luedtke *et al* 1987).

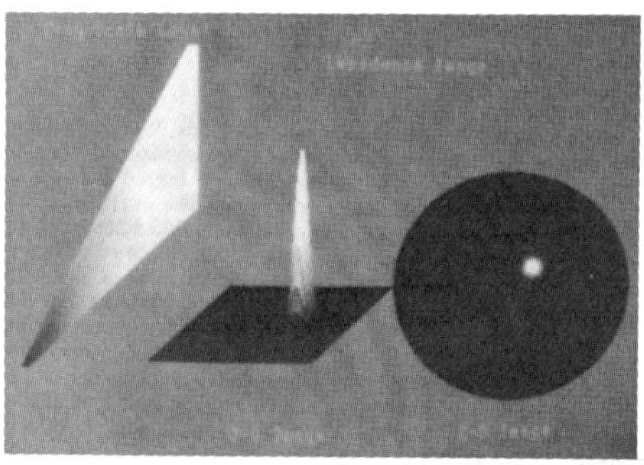

Figure 13.7 The reconstructed image of the cross section of the leg. The bright region in the image is the region of low resistivity (Luedtke *et al* 1987).

For patients suffering from DVT, the thrombi in the leg would impede the blood flow, which implies that the creation of a low-impedance region will be slower. Images taken at two different times, one before and one after the occurrence of thrombosis, would, to a certain extent, help the physician detect the presence of these thrombi in the leg. Therefore, we could use dynamic imaging in detecting DVT. This method doesn't seem very useful, unless we can devise some means of obtaining quantitative information, like plots that can be obtained using venous occlusion plethysmography.

13.4 PULMONARY PERFUSION

Electrical impedance tomography could be used to determine the change in fluid volume within the lung, which could be related to the changes in the thoracic impedance. Lung tissue basically has two components—air (80%) and fluid (liquid)(5%). During maximal inspiration, the amount of air exceeds the amount of fluid inside the lungs, and hence the impedance is maximal; during maximal expiration, the amount of air decreases inside the lungs, which implies a decrease in the impedance. Therefore, any increase in the proportion of the fluid in the lungs would imply a significant drop in impedance. Pomerantz *et al* (1969) carried out experiments on humans and confirmed the relationship. The changes in electrical impedance can, therefore, be used as a means for detecting impending pulmonary edema.

Goldensohn and Zablow (1959) used a four-electrode method to correlate the volume of fluid in the lung and the transthoracic impedance. They placed two ECG electrodes, one on each wrist and passed a constant 10 kHz current between these electrodes. Two similar electrodes were placed farther up on each arm, and the voltage changes observed between the two. They compared the impedance changes and the respired volume by the method of least squares and found a linear relationship between the two.

In severe edema, the volume of interstitial fluid alone may increase by 0.12–0.2 liter (Harris *et al* 1987). There is at present no method for measuring the amount of water inside the lungs which is suitable for routine use. EIT is quite sensitive to changes in lung water, but cannot give any quantitative information. EIT can be used to image the effect of changes in lung volume. Henderson and Webster (1978) designed and built an impedance camera to obtain impedance images of the thorax. They used an array of 100 mutually guarding current-measuring electrodes, and used the 44 nonmeasuring electrodes as guards (15 mm diameter), all applied to the subject's back. They obtained the isoadmittance contour map shown in figure 1.2. Though the spatial resolution in this camera is limited, we can speculate that EIT could be used to obtain static images of the thorax, which could provide useful information about patients suffering from pulmonary edema. The 16 Ag/AgCl electrodes could be placed, equally spaced, all around the thorax (including the back). High-frequency current could be applied to all the electrodes simultaneously to obtain a desired current distribution (say, $\cos\theta$). The adaptive method (also called optimal current method) of data collection would be the best for this type of static image (see Section 8.6). The impedance image obtained with this type of data collection would have the maximal distinguishability. No *in vivo* images of the presence of fluid in the lungs have been obtained, but we believe that these could be obtained. Using EIT, theoretically, a spatial resolution of about 8% of the array diameter could be obtained, which implies a resolution of 2 cm within the thorax. The sensitivity to change is very good. Theoretically, a 2% decrease in lung tissue resistivity as blood perfuses the tissue during systole could be imaged (Brown and Barber 1987).

13.5 PULMONARY VENTILATION

Many investigators have demonstrated a high correlation between thoracic impedance change and volume of air breathed (Geddes and Baker 1989). Figure 13.8 is a typical record of ventilation and impedance variation from the thorax. To obtain these results, we injected a 50-kHz current of 5 mA through two tetrapolar electrodes (figure 10.4) placed at the level of the xiphoid process and along the midaxillary lines. The ventilation signal, top channel, was recorded by coupling a low torque potentiometer to the pulley suspending the bell of a spirometer. The impedance on the thorax, bottom channel, was recorded by amplifying the measured impedance after subtracting the baseline. The impedance variation is about 1% of the baseline impedance. In order to use the full range of the ADC, we subtracted the average baseline impedance from the varying impedance. Comparing two channels shows that there is a high correlation between the thoracic impedance and volume of breathed air. Baker and Geddes (1965) reported a fairly good linearity between impedance and volume changes. The relation between impedance and volume changes depends on the size of the subject and the location of the electrodes.

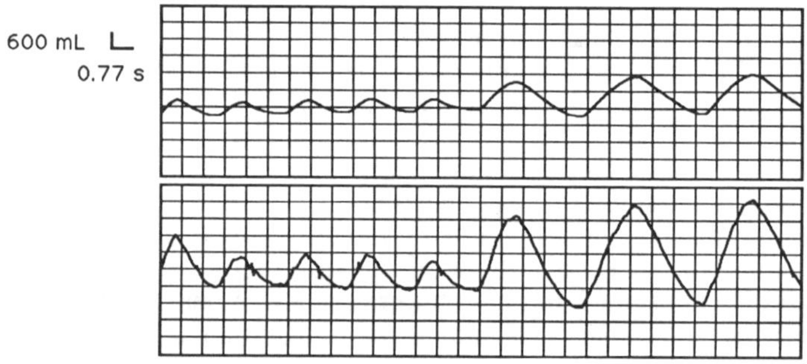

Figure 13.8 Top channel shows direct measurement of tidal volume recorded from a spirometer. Bottom channel is impedance variation across thorax using an arbitrary scale. Note the high correlation between thoracic impedance change and volume of air breathed for different levels of ventilation.

Ideally we can use this linear relation to measure pulmonary ventilation by monitoring the thoracic impedance after calibrating the system by a spirometer (Kubicek *et al* 1964). Even though for long-term monitoring, this indirect measurement is simple and more convenient than using the spirometer, there are some practical problems. For example, most normal people are thoracic breathers in the upright position and abdominal breathers in the supine or prone position (Druz and Sharp 1981). Also during different stages of sleep, rapid eye movement (REM) and nonrapid eye movement (NREM), excursion of the chest wall and abdomen may vary and affect calibration (Gould *et al* 1988). Another big problem is the effect of body motion on the signal. Figure 13.9 shows the effects of body motions on the impedance recorded from two electrodes across the thorax. The subject did not move for the first two breaths and then started moving his upper body for four breaths. Then the subject was asked to stop breathing while continuing his body movement and when he started moving his arms the impedance variation went off scale.

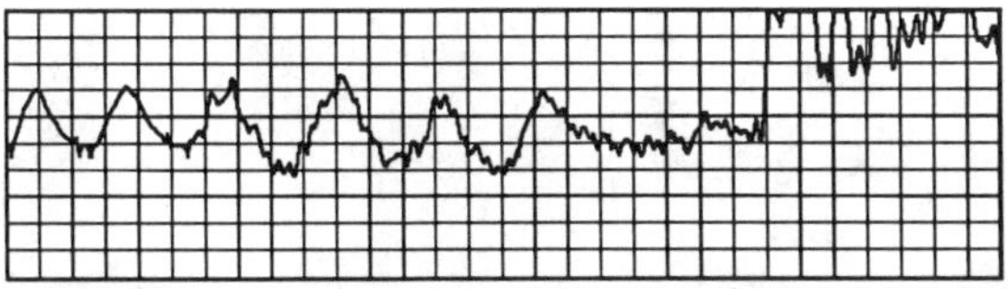

Figure 13.9 Recorded thoracic impedance for no movement, upper body movement, movement without breathing and moving arms.

During sleep, the body undergoes a variety of changes that complicate the measurement of lung volume using impedance. While normal adult tidal volume is 500 ml, during quiet periods of sleep, this may drop to 100 ml, then increase to 1000 ml. During some periods chest breathing may dominate, later, abdominal breathing may dominate. During REM sleep, the ribs move hardly at all. Sometimes paradoxical breathing causes the rib cage to move inwardly while the abdomen expands. Mild snoring causes changes in the configuration of chest wall. Blood shifts within the lung tissue can cause impedance changes to occur even when there is no change in lung volume. Different muscle groups may relax, which makes the remaining groups work harder. Finally, the body assumes a variety of positions during the night, each of which may have a different impedance/lung volume calibration.

Henderson and Webster (1978) obtained the isoadmittance contour map of the thorax by frontal plane imaging (see figure 1.2). It shows significant variations of resistivity within the thorax. Brown *et al* (1985) argue that the signals obtained from the impedance pneumograph are very large (approximately 1% of the baseline impedance), and therefore can be used to reconstruct EIT images. The resistivity of lung tissue changes within the range 10 to 20 Ω m from expiration to inspiration (Barber and Brown 1984). They used a 16-electrode technique, obtained impedance images from the two lungs, and found that these images could be separated.

Harris *et al* (1987) obtained a dynamic image of the lung. They used 16 Ag/AgCl electrodes, equally spaced, all around the thorax between the 2nd and 6th intercostal spaces. High-frequency current was applied between a pair of electrodes, and voltages measured between all other adjacent pairs. This process was repeated for all different drive pairs. In order to minimize artifacts from the cardiac cycle, they averaged about 40 data-collection cycles, which effectively increased the SNR. Each of the voltages measured was divided by the voltage obtained from a reference data set. The logarithm (ln) of this ratio was backprojected to obtain an image. All the backprojected images obtained were added and then filtered to obtain the final image. Figure 13.10 shows the different regions of resistivities (white is a region of high resistivity) which correspond to the changes in the lung volume. They also carried out experiments by placing electrodes at different levels (3, 4, 5) of the intercostal spaces, and obtained dynamic images.

The present methods for the measurement of the level of ventilation in the lungs use radioisotope lung scans, which are harmful. EIT can be used repeatedly without causing any harm to the patient. The EIT image can only give a cross-sectional view of the lung in a plane, unlike the radioisotope scans, which cover the entire lung.

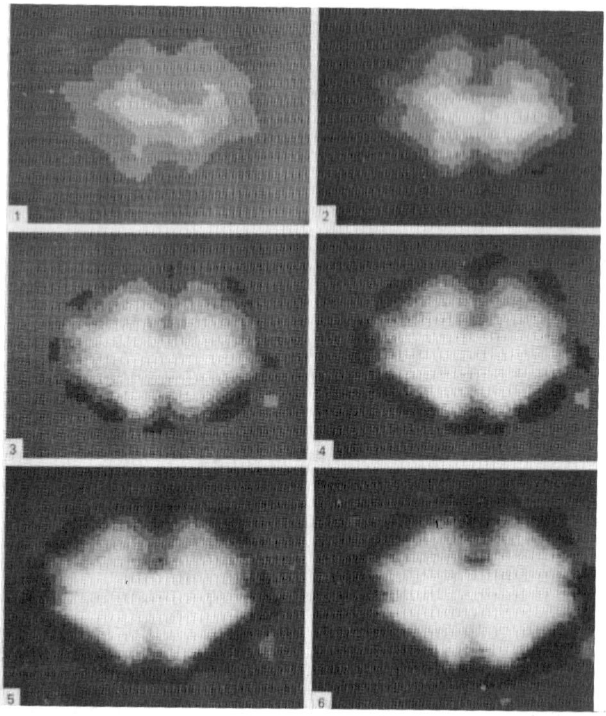

Figure 13.10 The changes in the lung volume during inspiration correspond to the changes in resistivity. The regions of high resistivity (white region) correspond to the two lungs (Harris *et al* 1987).

Static imaging would be very useful in detecting apnea. But the *a priori* knowledge of the exact position of the electrodes makes it extremely difficult to obtain static images.

Dynamic images obtained using EIT could be used to monitor infants who are prone to apneic episodes. A possible method would be to monitor continuously the change in thoracic impedance; if this change were below a certain threshold value, an alarm could sound (after about 10–15 s) for timely response and possible resuscitation. The next section describes currently used apnea monitors.

13.6 APNEA MONITORING

Apnea is cessation of breathing for more than 20 s, or ventilatory pause associated with cyanosis, marked pallor, hypotonia or bradycardia (American

Academy of Pediatrics 1978). Infants suffering from prolonged apnea are at risk of sudden infant death syndrome (SIDS). Apnea accounts for many deaths among prematurely born infants and we can prevent some of infant sudden deaths by detecting episodes of apnea. There are three types of apnea seen in infants; central, obstructive and mixed (Fleming 1983). Central apnea is disappearance or diminish of ventilatory effort which is because of a deficiency in respiratory control. In this type of apnea, respiratory muscles do not act and there is neither motion on the chest nor airflow. In obstructive apnea, ventilatory effort continues but the respiratory airway is blocked. In this case, there is no airflow but the chest has motion. Mixed apnea usually begins with an obstructive apnea and then is followed by central apnea because of fatigue, increase in carbon dioxide level and reduction of oxygen.

The most reliable and accurate apnea detection is using direct measurement of airflow. For example, spirometers measure the tidal volume, airflow sensors such as nasal thermistors detect the airflow and gas flowmeters measure rate and volume of the airflow. For long-term monitoring, these devices are inconvenient and not well tolerated. Nasal thermistors loose their sensitivity due to the moisture they absorb from airflow. Most of these devices are not easy to operate especially for home monitoring. For home monitoring, cost and simplicity are two important criteria as well as reliability.

Indirect methods monitor the effects of ventilation such as gross-body motion, chest-wall motion, chemical effects (O_2 and CO_2 level in blood or expired gases) and impedance variation of the chest wall. There are different configurations that sense the motion of the body or the chest wall. They all use pressure sensors such as piezoelectric sensors to detect body motions and fail to detect obstructive apnea reliably because they might identify body motion as ventilation regardless of existence of airflow. Some of these motion sensors are difficult to install and adjust. There are some devices such as oximeters which can determine the level of O_2 in blood. Apnea may be detected by low level of O_2 in blood. Reliability of these devices depends on how accurately they determine O_2 level and how fast apnea decreases O_2 level in blood. Another indirect method is measuring impedance variation on the chest wall which is related to the air volume in the lungs. The next section also addresses some of the problems and suggests using multiple electrodes which may improve the overall performance of impedance pneumography.

Impedance-based apnea monitors are the most commonly used devices for apnea detection. Figure 13.11 shows a typical configuration for an impedance-based apnea monitor. The device injects a small high-frequency current across the thorax through two electrodes. The current is in the range of 5 mA at a frequency of 50 to 100 kHz. Electrodes can be of the electrocardiographic (ECG) or carbon-loaded rubber type. Carbon-loaded rubber electrodes might be preferred over ECG electrodes because they are reusable and do not cause irritation. Air volume variation in the lungs modulates the voltage drop across the thorax which is measured by the same electrodes. The monitor demodulates the voltage drop and uses analog or digital methods to identify ventilatory signals. If there is no ventilatory signal for a preset period of time (selected by the user between 10 to 30 s) the device sets a warning alarm. The same two electrodes combined with an extra electrode can extract the ECG signal for heart rate monitoring and detecting bradycardia. Impedance-based apnea monitors are easy to operate and economical which make them suitable and practical for home monitoring. The next section describes reliability and some problems with these type of monitors.

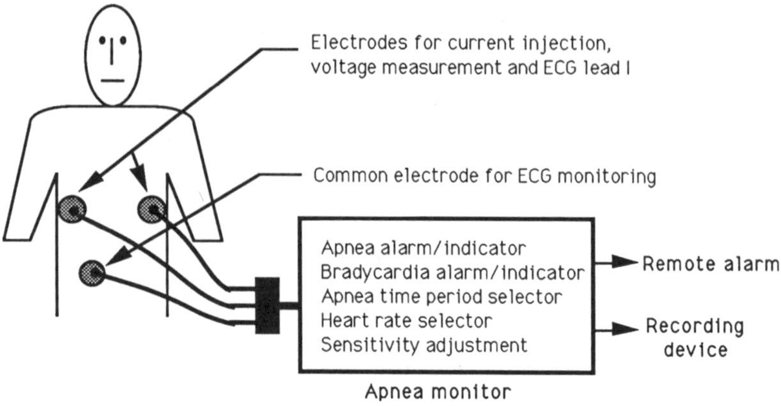

Figure 13.11 A typical home apnea monitor measures changes in impedance between electrodes placed on the left and right sides of the thorax.

Although impedance-based apnea monitors are the most commonly used devices especially for home monitoring, their performance is not satisfactory. Black *et al* (1978) studied the impact of the apnea monitor on family life. The study showed that home monitoring had numerous shortcomings. Most families experienced mechanical problems using the monitor at home. These problems included fragility of leads, electrode placement and sensitivity adjustment. Sensitivity adjustment is very important because low sensitivity causes too many false alarms and frustration of the family where as high sensitivity disables the device to distinguish motion artifacts from ventilation. These types of monitors usually fail to detect obstructive apnea because they register thoracic movements as ventilation. Warburton *et al* (1977) concluded that these types of apnea monitors are unsuitable for monitoring infants at risk for upper airway obstruction. Figure 13.12 shows a simulation of obstructive apnea after recording normal breaths. The subject occluded his airway but kept on contracting and relaxing his ventilatory muscles. Apnea monitors may identify these ventilatory efforts as breathing even though there is no airflow.

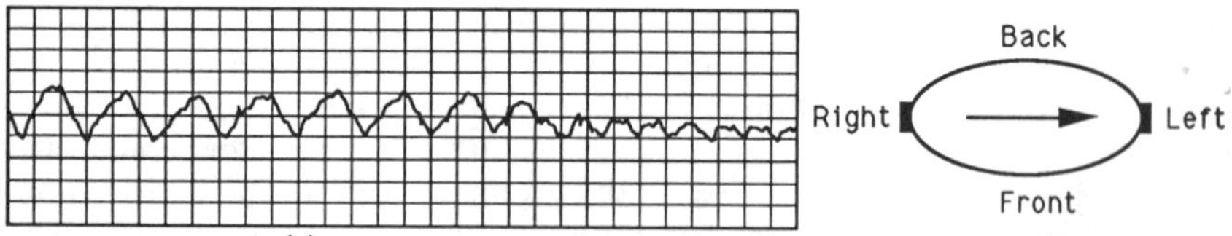

(*a*) (*b*)

Figure 13.12 (*a*) Small peaks at the end of the recording show ventilatory efforts although there is no airflow. (*b*) Electrodes were placed at the level of the xiphoid process and along the midaxillary lines. Arrow shows the direction of current flow.

To improve the performance of impedance-based monitors, we need to identify the main reason for the poor performance of these monitors and then look for potential solutions. These devices monitor the impedance variation across the thorax. The volume of the air in the lungs determines the resistivity of the lungs and therefore the thorax. There are other factors, beside lung resistivity, which change the thoracic impedance. Some of these factors are the change in the circumference of the thorax during ventilation, the change in the current pathway due to ventilation and the movement of the skin or body and the change in contact impedance of electrodes. It is important to determine the contribution of the lungs in changing the impedance of the thorax. Baker and Geddes (1966) measured the thoracic impedance at the xiphoid level of dead dogs and measured the current through different pathways. They found that only 4.7 percent of the total current was conducted through the lungs and 79.9 percent conducted through the posterior thoracic pathway. Albisser and Carmichael (1974) used a theoretical model to show that geometrical factors of chest circumference and interelectrode distance make significantly greater contributions to thoracic impedance change than lung resistivity variations.

It seems that volume change of the lungs yields a small contribution to the thoracic impedance change and other factors such as motion artifacts can easily mask the ventilation signal. One potential solution would be using more than two electrodes to direct the current into the lungs. This method could increase the contribution of the lungs to conducting the injected current and eventually the change in thoracic impedance. Figures 13.13(*a*) and (*b*) show the simulation of apnea after normal ventilation using four and eight electrodes respectively. We tried to keep all the conditions such as subject's position and amount of ventilation the same as in the case of using two electrodes (figure 13.12). We could obtain reasonable improvement by using multiple electrodes and a suitable current pattern. Figure 13.13 shows that for the multiple-electrode method, the signal from ventilation effort without airflow (obstructive apnea simulation) is less than that in the two-electrode method. Note that we could improve the recorded signal only for suitable current patterns such as the one shown in figure 13.13(*b*).

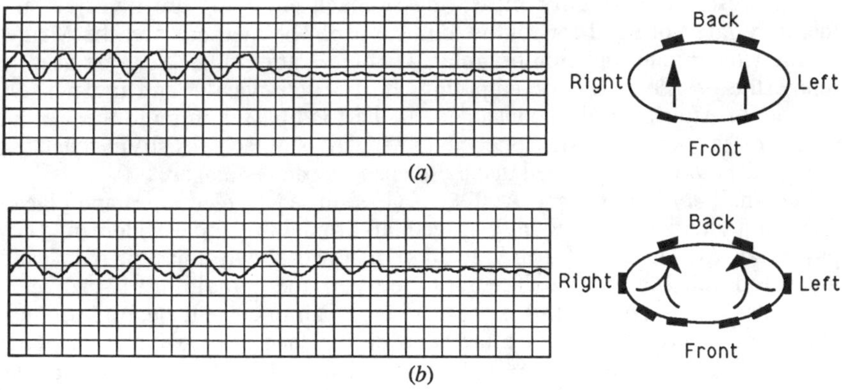

Figure 13.13 Recorded signal from multiple electrodes (RMS values) with obstructive apnea simulation. Electrode positions and current patterns are shown: (*a*) four electrodes (*b*) eight electrodes.

13.7 STOMACH EMPTYING

The rate of stomach emptying can be used to detect congenital heart diseases, gastroesophagal reflux and pyloric stenosis. It can also be used for studying the influence of the component parts of various types of food on gastric emptying, such as the fat proportion (Murphy *et al* 1987).

McClelland and Sutton (1985) used a tetrapolar arrangement to find changes in the impedance of the epigastrium (the upper middle region of the abdomen, located within the sternal angle). They used the electrode placement shown in figure 13.14. The subjects lay semisupine at approximately 45° with their legs stretched out before them. Adhesive Ag/AgCl electrodes were used, as they provided better electrode contact, and also reduced the baseline impedance from 20 Ω to 10–12 Ω. A 4 mA, 100 kHz AC current was passed between the input electrodes, and the changes in impedance measured between the recording electrodes. They measured impedance changes in the range 0.80 to 1.33 Ω, for different types of meals (600 ml).

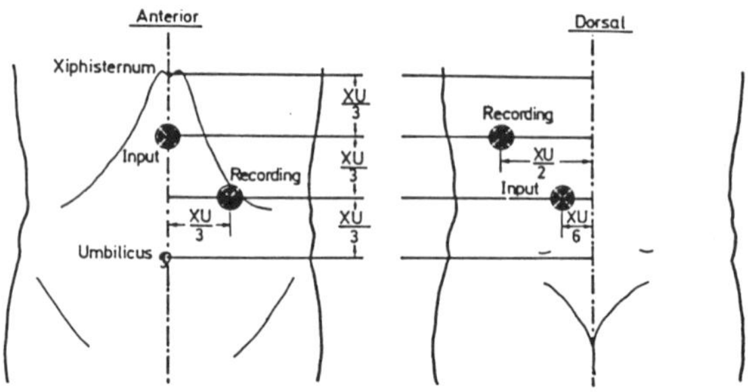

Figure 13.14 Standard electrode placement for measuring epigastric impedance (McClelland and Sutton 1985).

The present methods for measuring stomach emptying are invasive, and therefore, are not ideal for routine clinical use. The methods are: the Marker dilution technique and Scintigraphy (Gamma Camera). EIT can be used to image the profile of gastric emptying. It is a noninvasive and inexpensive technique. After a meal is consumed, as the food passes through the various stages of the stomach and upper abdomen, the stomach resistivity changes. Mangnall *et al* (1987) showed that these changes can be imaged.

Mangnall *et al* (1987) and Avill *et al* (1987) used 16 electrodes and placed them in a circular array, equally spaced, all around the upper abdomen. They passed an AC current of 1 mA at 50 kHz between two adjacent pairs, and measured the potential differences between the remaining 13 adjacent electrodes. They repeated this process for each pair of current electrodes. Thus, they made 208 (= 16 × 13) measurements during each cycle, which took about 100 ms. A preprandial data set is first recorded, and all the next postprandial data sets are backprojected against the first data set to produce a cross-sectional dynamic image (Section 13.2). Figure 13.15 shows a sequence of images obtained by Avill *et al* (1987), before and after the consumption of a drink of

Oxo (a conductive drink). They also found that the profiles of stomach emptying were very similar to those obtained using the gamma camera and marker dilution technique. In order to inhibit the acid secretion into the stomach, they used 800 mg of cimetidine; acid secretion is believed to reduce the resistivity of gastric contents. EIT can also be used to measure the gastric acid secretion.

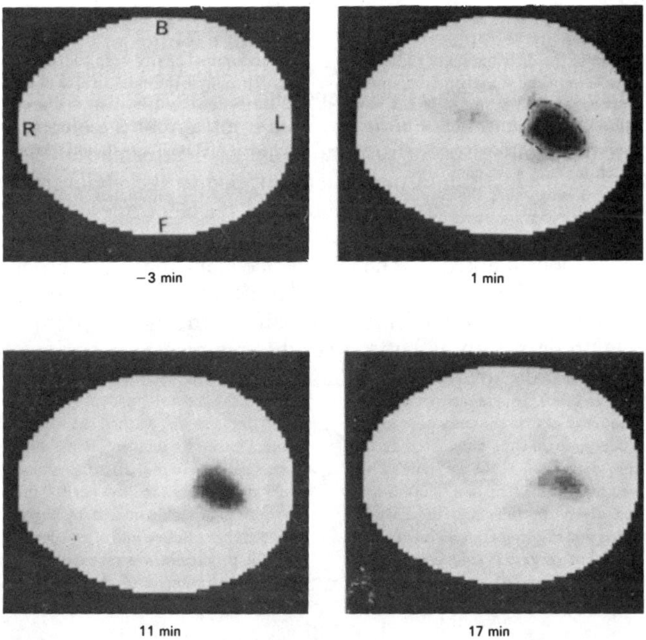

Figure 13.15 Sequence of images before and after the consumption of the drink Oxo (at different times), showing gastric emptying. The dark patches represent regions of decreased resistivity (Avill *et al* 1987).

13.8 BLADDER VOLUME

The measurement of bladder volume is important in the investigation of patients suffering from a disturbance of bladder fullness (micturition), which is defined as the urge to void. The problem of bladder fullness is very prevalent among the elderly, particularly elderly women. Also the urinary bladder may be paralyzed by spinal-cord injury. In the United States of America, there are about 5 million people who are incontinent, of which approximately 160000 are mentally retarded (Winfield *et al* 1988).

Ultrasonic imaging of the bladder is the most commonly used diagnostic procedure. The ultrasonic bladder sensor provides the user an external electric signal, which acts as an internal stimulus. The volume of urine is continuously monitored using this device, and when it reaches the threshold level, the user is alerted by an alarm. This method requires the patient to remain supine and immobile (Mineo 1986).

Denniston and Baker (1975) carried out experiments on mongrel dogs (all anesthetized) and found that the electrical impedance (measured using an Impedance Cardiograph, with a constant current source of 4 mA at 100 kHz) varied linearly with the volume of urine infused into the bladder. Doyle and Hill (1975) conducted experiments on humans, with male patients sitting upright on a commode and female patients lying on an examination couch. They found a linear decrease in impedance with the increase of the bladder volume.

The bladder lies on the outside of the abdominal cavity, and is near the front. When the bladder is full, it lies just beneath the skin, fat and muscle, between the *symphysis pubis* and the *umbilicus*. This implies that the electrodes should be placed in the front in order to obtain maximal information. Figure 13.16 shows a tetrapolar electrode arrangement applied to the abdominal skin. The electrodes placed farther away are the current (*I*) electrodes. High-frequency current is applied to these electrodes, and the corresponding voltage measured across the electrodes marked *V*. The impedance change gives a direct indication of the change in bladder volume. The optimal placement of the current electrodes can be estimated by finding the half-width angle, θ (figure 12.5). The tetrapolar electrode system is better than the two-electrode system, because it measures change only between the voltage electrodes (Section 3.5).

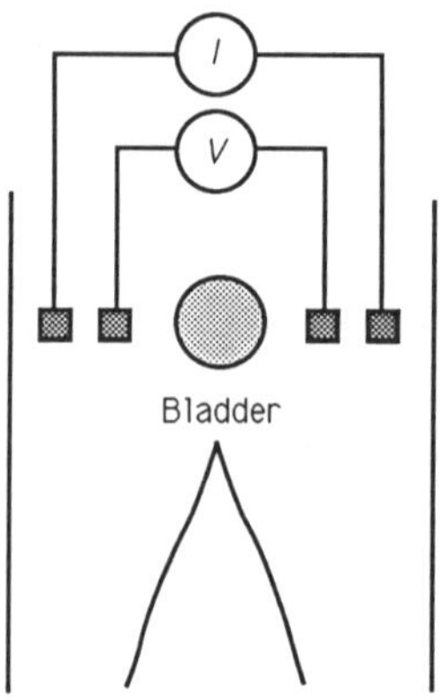

Figure 13.16 Typical tetrapolar electrode arrangement for measuring bladder fullness.

EIT, a noninvasive technique, could be used to monitor the urine accumulation in the bladder. Though no *in vivo* measurements have been made, the following electrode placement is possible. The eight Ag/AgCl (spot) electrodes are placed in the same plane longitudinally (figure 13.17). Current (~5 mA) at 50 kHz is passed between two electrodes and voltages measured between the remaining electrodes. A linear array (Section 8.7) would be good, in order to get a better current distribution near the bladder. A better method would be injecting current through all the electrodes rather than two (as in the adaptive method). The voltage change with respect to the bladder volume change would be the greatest in this case, implying a better distinguishability (as opposed to other data collection methods). The SNR is also maximal in this case (see Section 10.7). As a guard voltage can only be defined to follow the voltage of a single electrode, it is worth noting that they are not useful in this type of measurement using eight electrodes. Moreover, guards help control the current distribution, and in the case of measuring bladder fullness, we need a high current density near the bladder.

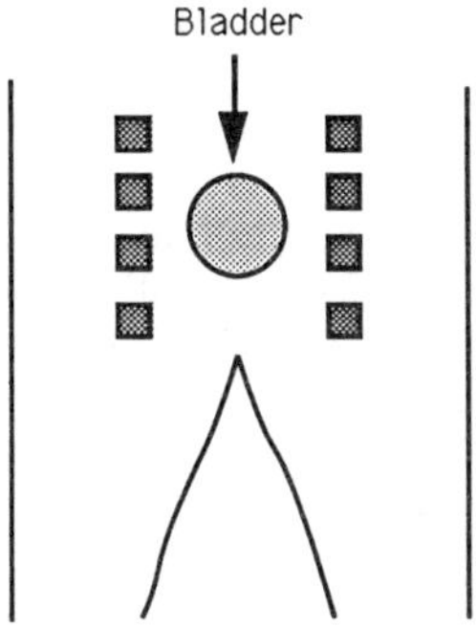

Figure 13.17 A possible 8-electrode placement for EIT for measuring bladder fullness. The electrodes are placed vertically because the bladder moves vertically as it fills.

The kidney excretes urine into the bladder. It would be useful to generate an impedance image of the kidney to diagnose kidney degeneration when disease is present. It may be difficult to obtain adequate spatial resolution from surface electrodes. In this case it might be possible to introduce a catheter containing one or more electrodes. With these located within the kidney, together with surface electrodes, it might be possible to improve spatial resolution in the immediate vicinity of the kidney.

13.9 BREAST TISSUE ANALYSIS

The detection of soft tissue lesions such as cysts and tumors is particularly important in breast tissue analysis, for the detection of malignancies in the breast. With the presently available methods, it is difficult to detect these lesions (Dawids 1987). EIT seems to be one possibility to tackle such a clinical problem. Fricke and Morse (1926) showed that the dielectric constant in the breast would change, if a tumor were present. Also, the highly vascularized tissue surrounding a tumor will have a low resistivity, which contrasts with the avascular tissue of the tumor; this change in resistivity (due to the growth of a tumor) could be sensed by EIT.

Skidmore *et al* (1987) have developed a data collection system for gathering electrical impedance measurements from the human breast. Figure 13.18 shows the electrode placement ring. They used 16 electrodes to completely encircle the human breast, and to maintain good contact they used gel. Using a programmable multiplexer system, they selected a pair of drive (current) electrodes, and used a 1 mA peak-to-peak 90 kHz sinusoidal current, and measured the respective voltages between the remaining electrodes to obtain the impedance values. No *in-vivo* images have been obtained so far, but the image reconstruction algorithms are in progress, which might make use of this computer-controlled data collection system. Static imaging is a possibility in this case, as the positions of the electrodes are known *a priori*. A lowering of the resistivity would indicate the presence of a tumor. This could be observed in the image obtained. The spatial resolution of this type of system is about 10–15% of the array diameter. Because the electrodes are attached to the periphery of the ring, the system would have a very low spatial resolution at the center, and a relatively higher spatial resolution at the periphery (near the circumference). This method doesn't seem very useful because of the poor spatial resolution for two-dimensional phantoms. Brown and Seagar (1985) claim that the achievable resolution for a 128-electrode system is about 1.5% of the array diameter (for two-dimensional phantoms), though not as good as that of X-ray CT or MRI systems.

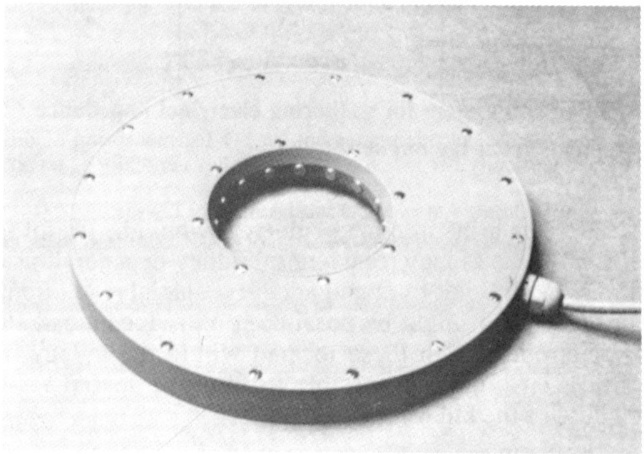

Figure 13.18 Electrode placement ring for breast tissue analysis (Skidmore *et al* 1987).

13.10 HYPERTHERMIA MONITORS

The need to measure the temperature deep within the tissues plays an important role in the detection and treatment of cancer. The present techniques are invasive, in which the thermocouples, thermistors or optical fibers are implanted in the patient to obtain the temperature profile within the body. There exists a need to develop a noninvasive technique.

EIT has been shown to respond to temperature changes in the tissues (Griffiths *et al* 1985). Conway (1987) performed experiments using a 150 mm diameter agar phantom. He placed 16 electrodes symmetrically around the phantom, sent in a low current at 50 kHz between the drive pairs, and measured the potential differences between all other adjacent pairs. He then heated the surface of the phantom (for about 10 min) using a microwave applicator. A thermocouple was also placed just below the agar surface, in order to correlate the resistivity (obtained from EIT) and the temperature data (obtained from the thermocouple). He obtained dynamic images, and found a temperature resolution better than 1°C. Figure 13.19 shows the variation of conductivity (for EIT) and temperature (for thermocouple) with time, with electrodes placed in a circle on the planar surface of the back. He performed a similar experiment on the scapular region of a volunteer, and found many image artifacts.

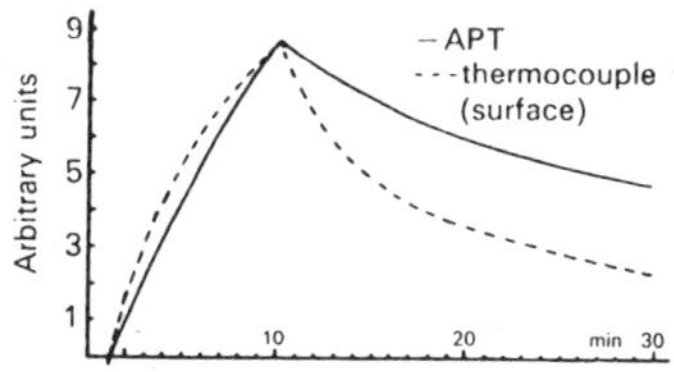

Figure 13.19 The variation of conductivity (for EIT or APT) and temperature (for thermocouple) with time, of the agar phantom heated with a microwave applicator (Conway 1987).

The temperature coefficient of electrical conductivity of tissue is about +2%/°C, which is very large compared to the X-ray absorption coefficient (in CT), which changes only by 0.04%/°C (Griffiths and Ahmed 1987b). A temperature increase, can, therefore, be deduced from a change in conductivity occurring during a hyperthermia treatment. Griffiths and Ahmed (1987b) used 16 electrodes, with the drive and voltage pairs selected using four 16-channel multiplexers. They required about 8 s to collect the data. They followed the same reconstruction principle as described in Section 13.2, except for the fact that they included an extra term (like a normalizing factor), which took into account the changes already made to the pixels in the band by previous backprojections. An initial data set was first collected (before heating), and all the other data sets collected after heating were related to the initial one. If V_1 and V_2 are the initial and final potential differences, then their ratio is backprojected according to the following formula:

$$\sigma_i' = \sigma_i \, (V_1/V_2)(1/\prod_j^N \sigma_j)^{1/N} \tag{13.8}$$

$$\ln\sigma_i' = \ln\sigma_i + \ln(V_1/V_2) - (1/N) \sum_j^N \ln\sigma_j \tag{13.9}$$

where σ_i and σ_i' = initial and updated values of the electrical conductivity in the ith pixel. N = total number of pixels.

Equation (13.9) can be rewritten (in a simplified notation) as

$$s_i' = s_i + \ln(V_1/V_2) - (1/N) \sum_j^N s_j \tag{13.10}$$

where $s_i'(s_i) = \ln\sigma_i'(\sigma_i)$.

The reconstruction starts by setting all pixels in the image to $s = 0$. The above procedure is then carried out iteratively. They finally used the following formula to smooth the image (process called spatial filtering):

$$s_i' = 0.5s_i + 0.073(s_1 + s_2 + s_3 + s_4) + 0.052(s_5 + s_6 + s_7 + s_8) \quad (13.11)$$

where subscripts 1 to 4 represent the four nearest neighbors, and 5 to 8, the four next nearest.

They performed *in vivo* measurements on the thigh of a volunteer with the 16 electrodes encircling the thigh, 18 cm above the knee, and the leg held in a horizontal position. They used a thermotherapy machine to deliver 13.56 MHz for about 6 min, and could obtain images while heating and cooling. A thermocouple was also used to monitor the temperature. The images show that EIT can be used effectively for the measurement of temperature during the treatment of carcinogenic cells.

13.11 TOTAL BODY WATER (TBW) AND BODY FAT

The measurement of human body composition would be of great help in determining the extent of malnutrition, or any other nutritional deficiencies that may go unnoticed. Body fluid change is very important for patients undergoing hemodialysis, or being treated for severe burns or any condition where the fluid balance is in question (Patterson *et al* 1988). The present direct methods include densitometry, anthropometric measurements, ultrasound, CT scan and many others. It has been shown that bioelectric impedance can be used to determine TBW, which is based on the electrical impedance plethysmography principle. The lean tissues (fat-free mass) are comprised mainly of electrolyte-containing water (73.2%), and therefore, conduct the applied electric current, whereas fat acts as an insulator and conducts little current. It is believed that these two compartments act in parallel, and therefore, the impedance of the body is mainly controlled by the lean-tissue component (Kushner and Schoeller 1986). It is well known that for a constant signal frequency, the impedance is related to the length and cross-sectional area of the conductor,

$$Z = \frac{\rho^* L}{A} \quad (13.12)$$

where Z = complex impedance (Ω), ρ^* = complex resistivity (Ω m) = $[1/(\sigma + j\omega\varepsilon\varepsilon_0)]$, L = length of the conductor (m) and A = conductor cross-sectional area (m^2).

Assuming that the lean tissue compartment is cylindrical, and that its volume is V, equation (13.12) can be written as

$$V = \frac{\rho^* L^2}{Z}. \quad (13.13)$$

Notice that Z, here, has both resistive and reactive components of a series model ($Z = (R^2 + X_C{}^2)^{1/2}$). Lukaski *et al* (1985) hypothesize that the magnitude of X_C is small relative to R, and that R is a better prediction of Z than is X_C. Similarly, ρ (= $1/\sigma$) is a better prediction of ρ^*. Equation (13.13) can therefore be written as

$$V = \frac{\rho L^2}{R}. \tag{13.14}$$

They used the tetrapolar electrode arrangement, with the subjects lying in a supine position. Note that in such an arrangement, the leg, the trunk and the arm are in series and therefore, the total resistance R is the sum of the three ($R = R_L + R_T + R_A \cong R_L + R_A$). A current of 800 μA at 50 kHz was introduced at the distal electrodes of the hand and foot, and the voltage drop was measured by the proximal electrodes. All the measurements were made 2 h after eating and within 30 min of voiding. The impedance (Z) was then calculated and hence the total body water (TBW). The lean body mass (LBM), also known as the fat-free mass (FFM), has been shown to be inversely related to R, and is given by the following relation (McDougall and Shizgal 1986):

$$\text{LBM} = \frac{16.4 + 0.61(\text{Ht})^2}{R} \quad (\text{kg}) \tag{13.15}$$

where Ht = height of the subject (cm).

The body fat (BF) is given by

$$\text{BF} = \text{BM} - \text{LBM} \quad (\text{kg}) \tag{13.16}$$

where BM = body mass (kg).

Lukaski *et al* (1985), Kushner and Schoeller (1986) and McDougall and Shizgal (1986) have observed good correlation between bioelectric impedance and densitometry, TBW and total body potassium determination.

For patients undergoing hemodialysis, the weight change due to the fluid change (as a result of hemodialysis), is related to the change in impedance, and is given by the following equation (Patterson *et al* 1988):

$$\Delta W_i = \frac{K(\text{Ht})^2(Z_{i\text{I}} - Z_{i\text{F}})}{Z_{i\text{I}} Z_{i\text{F}}} \tag{13.17}$$

where i = region of measurement: L (legs), T (trunk) or A (arms), ΔW_i = weight change due to fluid change, $Z_{i\text{I}}$ = initial impedance of the ith region, $Z_{i\text{F}}$ = final impedance of the ith region and K = proportionality constant depending on the resistivity of the fluid removed and on geometric factors ($K_A = 0.114$; $K_L = 0.060$; $K_T = 0.0041$).

EIT could be used to measure the parameters mentioned above. No *in vivo* experiments have been performed to date, but it is believed that EIT would be of value. A possible 16-electrode arrangement for determining the LBM and BF would be the same as shown in figure 13.6, wherein the spot electrodes are equally spaced all around the circumference. A high-frequency (50 kHz) current of magnitude 5 mA is applied between the drive pairs and the voltages measured between all the other adjacent electrodes. The ratio of the resistivity of fat to muscle is approximately 5:1. This high contrast in resistivity between fat and muscle should make them discernible in the image (theoretically). Figure 13.20 shows a speculated EIT image, showing the fat, muscle and bone. The spatial resolution of the image would not be very good. Retroperitoneal fibrosis is a condition in which the fat tissue is replaced by thickened connective tissue. Dawids (1987) conjectures that it may be possible to detect this with EIT. Presently, there is no technique available for detecting this type of fibrosis.

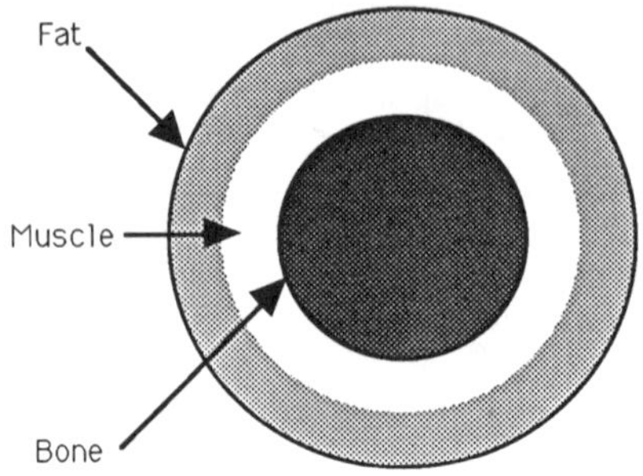

Figure 13.20 A typical image of the arm (having electrode positions as in figure 13.6), expected of EIT. Dark area shows high resistivity. (Typical values of resistivities: Fat, $\rho_f = 25$ Ω m; Muscle, $\rho_m = 1.5$ Ω m; Bone, $\rho_b = 166$ Ω m).

For measuring body water, a possible 16-electrode arrangement would be to place 16 spread out electrodes on the front and back of the trunk (where body water accumulates). We would need a three-dimensional model to measure both in-phase and reactive components at multiple frequencies. For patients undergoing hemodialysis, an initial frame of data would first be obtained before the start of the hemodialysis. Any subsequent data would then be backprojected on the initial set of data to obtain the dynamic image due to the changes in the body fluid volume.

13.12 MONITORING FRACTURE HEALING

Limb fractures are associated with large changes of electrical characteristics in the plane of the fracture which revert to normal during the healing process. Kulkarni *et al* (1989) used impedance imaging techniques to measure and image the spatial distribution of changes in resistivity during the healing process. It is known that there is suddenly a highly conductive region in the plane of the fracture subsequent to the occurrence of a diaphyseal fracture. Then, during the process of healing, the region recovers the normal electrical characteristics as the fracture hematoma is organized to form a dense mass of bone.

Kulkarni *et al* (1989) used 16 Ag/AgCl strip electrodes placed equidistantly on 25 mm wide elastic electrode belts. They used the backprojection method with 10 kHz 1 mA injection current. Figure 13.21 shows an image of a healed fracture. The two-dimensional impedance imaging technique is useful in impedance osteography since the region of interest is large and limb is axially symmetric.

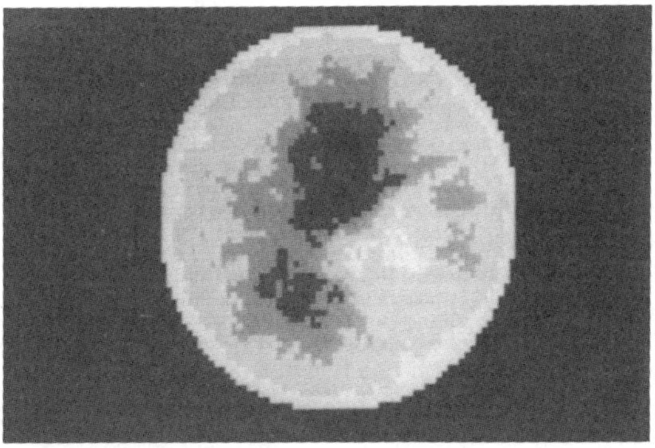

Figure 13.21 EIT image of a healed fracture (Kulkarni *et al* 1989).

13.13 BRAIN IMAGING

Impedance changes within the head have been studied using two- and four-electrode measurement methods but have yielded limited diagnostic capabilities. McArdle *et al* (1989) used the backprojection method with the Sheffield system using 16 electrodes to image the resistivity changes of the adult brain during the cardiac cycle. They found that the ECG-gated images were consistent for the same subject showing increases in conductivity following cardiac systole but that there were differences among 12 adult subjects.

They observed increasing conductivity at systole in a sequence of reconstructed images. The changes usually occurred in the central half/two thirds of the image with a peripheral annulus of lower activity. The amplitude of the changes was between 0.05% and 0.1%. These changes were recorded by averaging 500 cardiac cycles in order to reduce the system noise level. From a simulation study using an analytic model, they reported that the effect of the skull is to reduce sensitivity and causes some centripetal distortion. They believe that they can image the resistivity changes within the skull and that they are not just observing the backprojection of scalp blood flow into the center of the image. However, further research is required to explain the direction and amplitude of the observed changes and the wide variations among subjects in the images.

13.14 STUDY QUESTIONS

13.1 Give the most commonly used equation for measuring cardiac output using electrical impedance and define all terms.

13.2 Suggest a method for using EIT to measure cardiac output.

13.3 Describe the electrode placement and results obtained, when using EIT to measure cerebral hemodynamics.

13.4 Describe the electrode placement and results obtained, when using EIT to measure venous occlusion plethysmography.

13.5 Suggest the electrode placement, method of attachment and possible results from using EIT to measure pulmonary edema.

13.6 Describe the electrode placement and results obtained, when using EIT to measure pulmonary ventilation.

13.7 Estimate the spatial resolution and impedance magnitude resolution, when using EIT to measure the rate of stomach emptying.

13.8 Sketch and describe the electrode placement and method of attachment for a possible system to measure bladder volume.

13.9 Sketch the cross section of breast, show the current lines, and indicate the spatial sensitivity for detecting an object as a function of radius for EIT.

13.10 Give the sign and magnitude of resistivity change of tissue as a function of temperature as used in EIT hyperthermia monitors.

13.11 Explain how it is possible to measure body fluid and body fat using EIT.

13.12 What factors can change the calibration of an impedance pneumograph?

13.13 Explain how an impedance-based apnea monitor works and why it may fail to detect obstructive apnea.

13.14 What are the advantages and disadvantages of impedance pneumography?

13.15 Under what conditions could the multiple-electrode method improve the performance of apnea monitors?

13.16 Why is the sensitivity adjustment important for apnea monitors?

13.17 What are the problems associated with impedance-based apnea monitors?

14

Geophysical Prospecting

Sudhakar Bhat

Chapter 13 describes the many applications of electrical impedance tomography that have been used in the medical field. Lytle and Dines (1978) also have shown that the electrical resistivity technique can be used in geophysical prospecting to determine the subsurface resistivity distribution. Practical applications include hydrology, location of ore bodies and deposits of coal, sand or gravel, seismology studies, *in situ* coal gasification and many others (Lytle *et al* 1974). The major drawback of this resistivity technique is its low SNR. In other words, it has large sensitivity to minor changes in conductivity near the surface. The practical difficulty involved in dragging the electrodes along the surface makes this technique unsuitable for oil prospecting (Telford *et al* 1976).

14.1 GEOPHYSICAL MEASUREMENTS

Electrical impedance well logging is usually used in petroleum exploration to identify potential reservoir rocks, and determining their porosity and permeability and the nature of the fluids present. A commonly used method for recording electrical resistivity logs is the single electrode resistance logs, wherein a single electrode is lowered into a well on the end of an insulated length of wire. Low-frequency current (usually less than 60 Hz) is injected, and the potential difference between the in-hole electrode and an electrode located at the surface is recorded, and the resistance obtained is a function of the resistivity of the material surrounding the electrode.

The power sources used for making resistivity measurements may be either DC or low frequency AC, preferably less than 60 Hz. Because of the short life of the batteries, low-frequency AC is preferred. The two-electrode technique for determining the resistivity distribution of anomalies beneath the earth's surface is not common because the electrode contact impedance introduces large errors (Section 3.4). Thus the four-electrode technique is used. Two electrodes are used as current electrodes (or transmitters), and the other two as the voltage electrodes (or receivers). Figure 14.1(*a*) shows a typical four-electrode arrangement. The difference in potential between V_1 and V_2 is (Telford *et al* 1976)

$$\Delta V = \frac{rI/(2\pi)}{(1/r_1 - 1/r_2) - (1/r_3 - 1/r_4)} \tag{14.1}$$

where r_1, r_2, r_3 and r_4 are shown in figure 14.1(a).

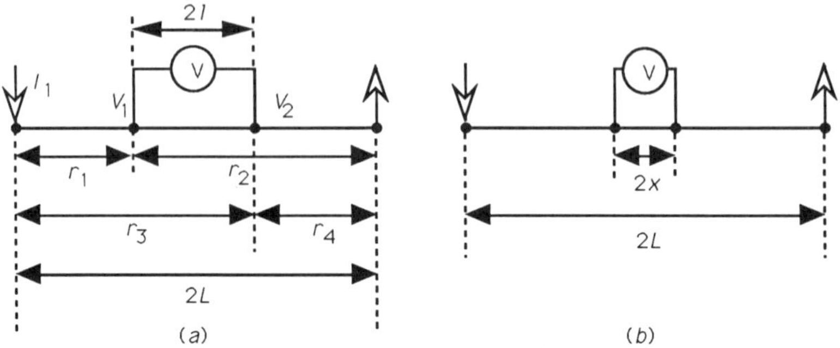

Figure 14.1 Different types of four-electrode arrays. (a) Wenner array; uniformly spaced. (b) Schlumberger array; widely spaced current electrodes. $2L$ is the total length of the array.

Figure 14.2 shows the equipotential and current flow-lines for two point sources of current. The contact impedance is a potential problem for small current electrodes, as the current density would be maximal in the vicinity of these electrodes, thereby creating a high potential gradient. Therefore, it is advisable to use large electrodes. These electrodes (known as probes), are about 100 to 150 mm long (Lytle *et al* 1974). Figures 14.1(a), (b), (c) show a few of the typical four-electrode arrays (Inman *et al* 1973). Current is injected between the electrodes marked I, and voltage measured across the electrodes marked V. The apparent resistivity of the earth (ρ) can then be determined from the ratio (V/I), and the geometrical arrangement of the electrodes. By moving this array along the earth's surface, and noting the changes in the resistivity, if any, we can detect subsurface objects, and relate these to geological structures. Lytle *et al* (1974) argue that it is possible to determine the presence of complex anomalies (with different regions having different resistivities as in a nonhomogeneous subsurface).

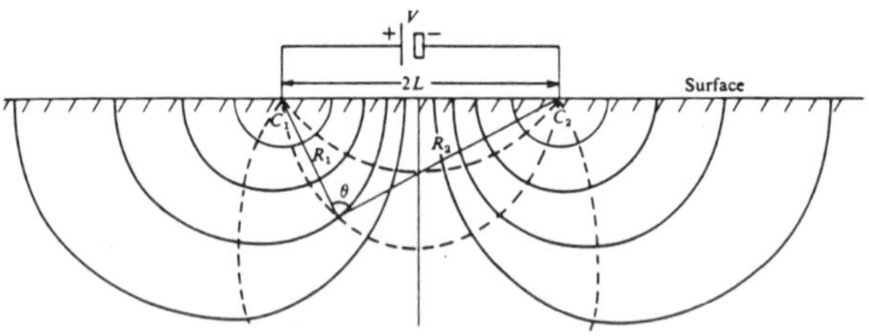

Figure 14.2 Equipotential and current flow-lines for two point sources of current (Telford *et al* 1976).

14.2 ELECTRODE ARRAYS

Figures 14.1(*a*), (*b*) show the most popular electrode arrays which are called *Wenner* and *Schlumberger* arrays. In the *Wenner* array (figure 14.1(*a*)), the electrodes are uniformly spaced, and $r_1 = r_4 = a$, and $r_2 = r_3 = 2a$. Thus the apparent resistivity follows from equation (14.1):

$$\rho_a = \frac{2\pi a \Delta V}{I}. \qquad (14.2)$$

This particular arrangement is often quite inconvenient for field work (Telford *et al* 1976). For depth exploration, the electrode distances are increased about a fixed center. For lateral exploration, the spacing between the electrodes is fixed, and all four electrodes are moved along a line. In the *Schlumberger* array, the current electrodes are spaced much further apart than the potential electrodes. The electrodes are placed symmetrically as shown in figure 14.1(*b*). Here, $r_1 = (L - l)$, $r_2 = (L + l)$, $r_3 = (L + l)$, and $r_4 = (L - l)$. The apparent resistivity (for $L \gg l$) is then

$$\rho_a = \frac{\pi L^2 \Delta V}{2lI}. \qquad (14.3)$$

In depth probing, the potential electrodes remain fixed, while the current electrode spacing is expanded symmetrically about the center. This method is more convenient than the *Wenner* type of array, because in this case only two electrodes move.

Figure 14.3 shows a two-dimensional cylindrical anomaly, having its axis parallel to the surface of the earth. This could be a mineral deposit. For probing such deposits, low-frequency electric current methods are used. The voltages are measured for different values of the distance x from the origin. The variation of the voltage V with distance x , i.e., $V = V(x)$, can be related to the presence of the anomaly. The ideal current electrode spacing, which is independent of the conductivity of the anomaly, can be found using figure 14.3. From the ratio of the radius of the cylindrical anomaly (r) and the distance of the center of the anomaly to the earth's surface (h), we determine the ideal half-width from figure 11.3 (Seagar and Bates 1985). The following example will clarify the point. Assume a circular cylindrical object having a radius of 2 m and with the center 4 m below the earth's surface. With $r/h = 0.5$, the ideal half-width per unit depth is $s/h = 0.87$. Therefore, the ideal full electrode separation for a 4 m depth is 6.96 m.

Wexler *et al* (1985) modeled the use of an 8 × 8 grid (i.e., 64 electrodes) over the earth's surface to obtain the conductivity distributions under the earth's surface. They introduced a current between two electrodes, and measured the voltages between a reference electrode and each of the other remaining electrodes. These measured surface voltage differences are related to the conductivity distribution underground. They initially made a guess of the conductivity distribution, and then calculated the voltage distribution throughout the region. They used the difference between the measured and the calculated potentials to update the conductivity estimate (see Section 10.6).

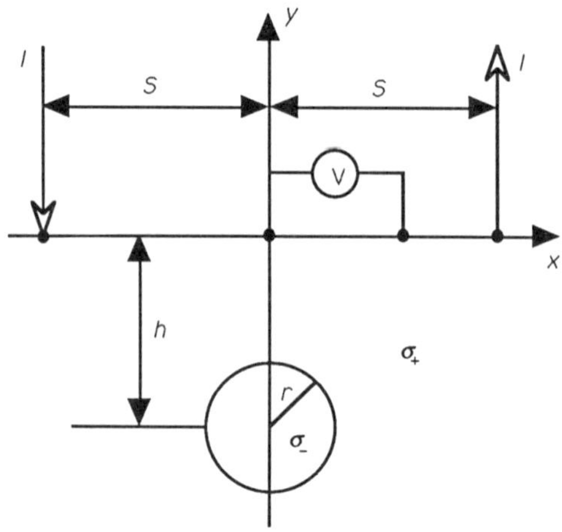

Figure 14.3 Cylindrical anomaly of radius r at depth h. $2s$ is the current-electrode separation; σ_- is the conductivity of the anomaly, and σ_+ is the conductivity of the surrounding earth (Seagar and Bates 1985).

Powell *et al* (1987) proposed that subsurface imaging is possible with a linear array of electrodes. Figure 8.6 shows the equipotential lines generated using a linear array of electrodes. They carried out experiments using a linear array, and found encouraging results. They placed 16 brass electrodes screwed through the Plexiglas wall of a tank of saline. They placed two spheres in the saline (the spheres had different resistivities from that of saline). They used the equipotential method (simple backprojection), as described in Section 10.4, and obtained the image. They could easily distinguish the two objects, but found an image artifact in the shape of an arc between them.

From Wexler's model, we could speculate that EIT could be used to image these subsurface profiles. Sixteen electrodes would be placed on the ground in a linear fashion. A 5 mA current would be injected into two electrodes, and voltages measured between the voltage reference and the remaining electrodes. This process would be repeated for all the different current pairs. This would give a total of 104 independent measurements. The maximal depth, D, up to which a body can be detected from the surface of the earth is called the limiting depth of detection (LDD) of the body (Roy and Rao 1977). LDD depends on the total length, L of the array. Powell *et al* (1987) have shown that, for homogeneous earth, the LDD is approximately equal to $0.5L$. In other words, the sensitivity (in terms of appreciable changes in estimated resistivity, due to different anomalies) of the linear array falls off rapidly with increasing depth, and therefore, this method can be used only to detect objects that are less than half the array length deep (see figure 8.7).

Traveltime tomography determines acoustic, seismic or electromagnetic wave speed distribution from first arrival traveltime data. Berryman (1989) developed a weighted least–square method which minimizes the predicted and measured traveltime data. He also imposed the variational constraints which guarantee that any optimal solution of the inverse problem lies in a convex region of the model space. Berryman (1990) developed a modified version of a damped least-squares algorithm whose correction step at each iteration is in the direction of the damped least–squares solution, but the size of the step is determined by the location of the point having the minimal number of feasibility violations in the direction of the step. He claimed that these techniques could also be applied in EIT reconstruction.

14.3 CORE SAMPLES

EIT can also be used to image and analyze the interior of a core sample. The core sample could be either square or cylindrical and the 16 electrodes could be placed all around the sample, equally spaced. The frequency of the current applied depends on the maximal characteristic spatial dimension, s, of the core sample, and the propagation constant, k, in the sample, and it is such that $|ks| < 0.01$ (Dines and Lytle 1981, Lytle *et al* 1974). By definition,

$$k = (\omega^2 \mu \varepsilon - \omega \mu_0 \sigma)^{1/2} \tag{14.4}$$

where $\omega = 2\pi f$; μ = permeability of the sample, ε = permittivity of the sample, σ = conductivity of the sample.

For nominal core samples, this typically means frequencies less than 1 kHz can be used. Lytle and Dines (1978) obtained conductivity profiles within computer models of square core samples, and could distinguish between regions of conductivities.

A dynamic image, obtained using EIT, could be useful to detect any underground chemical leakage. The chemicals might introduce a marked change in the resistivity, which could be easily resolved in the dynamic image.

14.4 STUDY QUESTION

14.1 Sketch the cross section of the use of EIT in geophysical prospecting and show the field line distribution. Show the electrode arrangement.

15

Active Groups and Companies

Sudhakar Bhat

This chapter includes the names and addresses of the various research groups and companies that have published in the field of Electrical Impedance Tomography in 1987 or later, or presented at the EEC workshops in Sheffield, England (1986) or Lyon, France (1987). Many active groups present their work each year at the Annual International Conference of the IEEE Engineering in Medicine & Biology Society, which publishes a proceedings describing this work.

15.1 ACTIVE RESEARCH GROUPS

The following is an alphabetical list of the names and addresses of persons and research groups, with their research interests, in the field of Electrical Impedance Tomography:

W R Breckon, M K Pidcock
Department of Computing and Mathematical Sciences
Oxford Polytechnic
Oxford OX3 0BP
UK
Data errors and reconstruction algorithms.

B H Brown, D C Barber, A D Seagar, N D Harris, A J Suggett, F J McArdle, R Pearce
Department of Medical Physics and Clinical Engineering, and Department of Medicine
Royal Hallamshire Hospital
Glossop Road
Sheffield S10 2JF
UK
Algebraic reconstruction technique, neighboring method, Sheffield system, applications of EIT.

S Dawids, L N Moesner*, O T Andersen*, J A Sorensen
Department of Engineering Design, Build. 421
*Electronics Institute, Build. 349
Technical University of Denmark
DK-2800 Lyngby
Denmark
Finite element model and image reconstruction, mathematical two-dimensional phantom model.

B M Eyuboglu
Center for Emerging Cardiovascular Technologies
Duke University
Durham, NC 27706
USA
Image variation during the cardiac cycle.

H Griffiths, Z Zhang
Department of Medical Physics and Bioengineering
University Hospital of Wales
Heath Park
Cardiff CF4 4XW
UK
Dual-frequency EIT, phantom made of resistors and capacitors.

R Guardo, C Boulay, B Murray, M Bertrand
Institut de Genie Biomedical
Ecole Polytechnique et Universite de Montreal
Montreal, Quebec
Canada
Resolution and image plane selectivity in EIT.

D S Holder, A R Gardner-Medwin
Department of Physiology
University College
London WC1E 6BT
UK
Imaging neuronal discharge and spreading depression in the brain.

M A Hussain, B Noble, B Becker
General Electric Research and Development Center
Schenectady, NY 12345
USA
Computer simulation of the inverse problem in EIT.

Y Z Ider
Department of Electrical and Electronic Engineering,
Middle East Technical University
Ankara, 06531
Turkey
Electrical impedance imaging system applicable to objects of arbitrary shape, but known boundary.

D Isaacson, D G Gisser*, J C Newell**
Department of Mathematics
*Department of Electrical and Computer Systems Engineering
**Department of Biomedical Engineering
Rensselaer Polytechnic Institute
Troy, NY 12180-3590
USA
Optimal current (adaptive) method, multiple electrode system.

J Jossinet, G Kardous
INSERM U281
151 Cours Albert Thomas
69003 Lyon
France
Sensitivity distribution in multielectrode systems.

Y Kim
Department of Electrical Engineering
University of Washington

Seattle, WA 98195
USA
Detection of DVT in human calf, microprocessor-based instruments and their applications, perturbation method.

R V Kohn
Courant Institute of Mathematical Sciences
251 Mercer Street
New York, NY 10012
USA
Reconstruction principles, relaxation method.

V Kulkarni, J M S Hutchison, I K Ritchie*, R B Chesney*, P Gibson*, J R Mallard
Department of Biomedical Physics and Bioengineering
*Department of Orthopaedics
University of Aberdeen and Grampian Health Board
Aberdeen AB9 2ZD, Scotland
UK
Monitoring fracture healing by impedance imaging.

H Kytomaa
Room 3-258A
MIT
77 Massachusetts Ave.
Cambridge, MA 02139
USA
Determination of two-phase flow in mineral slurry.

G L Lamont, J W Wright, D F Evans, L A Kapila
Department of Surgery
Queen's Medical Centre
Nottingham
UK
Detection of hypertrophic pyloric stenosis (HPS) in infants.

D Murphy, P Rolfe
Biomedical Engineering Centre
John Radcliffe Hospital
University of Oxford
Oxford
UK
Impedance imaging in the newborn.

J P O'Halloran
Department of Psychiatry and Human Behavior
University of California–Irvine
101 City Drive South
Orange, CA 92668
USA
Impedance imaging of the brain.

R Pallas-Areny, J Rosell
Division de Instrumentacion y Bioingenieria
ETSI Telecomunicacion
PO Box 30 002
08080 Barcelona
Spain
Error analysis in a parallel data acquisition system.

K Sakamoto
Faculty of Science and Technology
Sophia University

7-1 Kioi-Cho, Chiyoda-Ku
Tokyo 102
Japan
Reconstruction principles, physical phantoms.

Y Shi, B Rigaud, J Anah, J P Morucci, P M Marsill, G Mounie, R Bourret, M Granie
Unite de Recherche et de Transfert en Technologie Biomedicale
INSERM U 305
Hotel Dieu
31052 Toulouse Cedex
France
Data collection system, optimal control techniques and singular perturbation method for APT.

L Tarrasenko
Medical Engineering Unit
Department of Engineering Science
University of Oxford
Oxford OX1 3PJ
UK
Cerebral hemodynamics in the newborn using EIT.

J G Webster, W J Tompkins, P Hua, E J Woo, M R Akbarzadeh
Department of Electrical and Computer Engineering
University of Wisconsin–Madison
1415 Johnson Drive
Madison, WI 53706
USA
Finite element analysis, reconstruction algorithms and instrumentation, application for apnea monitoring and urinary bladder fullness.

A Wexler
Department of Electrical Engineering
University of Manitoba
Winnipeg, Manitoba R3T 2N2
Canada
Reconstruction algorithms, three-dimensional geophysical models, double constraint method.

W D Daily, T J Yorkey
L-156
Lawrence Livermore National Laboratory
Box 808
Livermore, CA 94550
USA
Reconstruction algorithms, core samples in geophysical prospecting.

15.2 ACTIVE COMPANIES

There is a company which builds EIT instruments and supplies these units (relating to specific applications) to medical personnel who are interested in taking the research to the next stage.

Wessex Medical Ltd.
Holmbush Estate, Midhurst
West Sussex GU29 9HX
UK

16

References

Akaike H 1974 A new look at statistical model identification *IEEE Trans. Automat. Contr.* **AC-19** 16–30

Albisser A M and Carmichael A B 1974 Factors in impedance pneumography *Med. Biol. Engng.* **12** 599–605

Alvarado F L 1977 Computational complexity of operations involving perfect elimination sparse matrices *Int. J. Computer Math.* **6** 69–82

American Academy of Pediatrics 1978 Task force on prolonged apnea *Pediatrics* **61** 651–2

Analog Devices 1989 *AD630 Balanced Modulator/Demodulator* (Norwood, MA: Analog Devices)

Association for the Advancement of Medical Instrumentation 1985 *Safe Current Limits for Electromedical Apparatus (ANSI/AAMI ES1-1985)* (Arlington, VA: AAMI)

Avill R, Mangnall Y F, Bird N C, Brown B H, Barber D C, Seagar A D, Johnson A G and Read N W 1987 Applied potential tomography: A new non invasive technique for measuring gastric emptying *Gastroenterology* **92** 1019–26

Baker L E and Geddes L A 1965 Quantitative evaluation of impedance spirometry in man. *Am. J. Med. Elect.* **4** 73–7

Baker L E and Geddes L A 1966 Transthoracic current paths in impedance spirometry. *Proc. Symp. Biomed. Eng.* 181–6

Barber D C and Brown B H 1984 Applied potential tomography *J. Phys. E: Sci. Instrum.* **17** 723–33

Barber D C and Brown B H 1986 Recent developments in applied potential tomography *Information Processing in Medical Imaging* ed S Bacharach (Dordrecht: Martinus Nijhoff) pp 446–62

Barber D C and Brown B H 1988a Errors in reconstruction of resistivity images using a linear reconstruction technique *Clin. Phys. Physiol. Meas.* **9 Suppl. A** 101–4

Barber D C and Brown B H 1988b Applied potential tomography—body shapes/static images UK patent application 8808969

Barber D C, Brown B H and Freeston I L 1983 Imaging spatial distributions of resistivity using applied potential tomography *Elec. Lett.* **19** 933–5

Barber D C and Seagar A D 1987 Fast reconstruction of resistive images *Clin. Phys. Physiol. Meas.* **8 Suppl. A** 47–54

Bard Y 1970 Comparison of gradient methods for the solution of nonlinear parameter estimation problems *SIAM J. Numer. Anal.* **7** 157–86

Berryman J G 1990 Stable iterative reconstruction algorithm for nonlinear traveltime tomography *Inverse Problems* in press

Berryman J G 1989 Weighted least-squares criteria for seismic traveltime tomography *IEEE Tran. Geoscience and Remote Sensing* **27** 302–9

Bertsekas D P and Tsitsiklis J N 1989 *Parallel and Distributed Computation* (Englewood Cliffs, NJ: Prentice-Hall)

Black L, Hersher L and Steinschneider A 1978 Impact of the apnea monitor on family life *Pediatrics* **62** 681–5

Brown B H 1983 Tissue impedance methods *Prog. Med. Environmental Phys.* **2** 85–110

Brown B H and Barber D C 1987 Electrical impedance tomography: the construction and application to physiological measurement of electrical impedance changes *Med. Prog. Tech.* **13** 69–75

Brown B H, Barber D C, Eyuboglu B M, Harris N D and McArdle F 1987 Electrical impedance imaging developed to image cardiopulmonary function *Proc. Annu. Int. Conf. IEEE Engineering in Medicine and Biology Society* **9** 1200–2

Brown B H, Barber D C and Seagar A D 1985 Applied potential tomography: possible clinical applications *Clin. Phys. Physiol. Meas.* **6** 109–21

Brown B H and Seagar A D 1985 Applied potential tomography: data collection problems *Proc. IEE Int. Conf. on Electric and Magnetic Fields in Medicine and Biology* 79–82

Brown B H and Seagar A D 1987 The Sheffield data collection system *Clin. Phys. Physiol. Meas.* **8 Suppl. A** 91–7

Burger H C and Dongen R 1961 Specific electrical resistance of body tissues *Phys. Med. Biol.* **5** 431–47

Burnett D S 1987 *Finite Element Analysis: from Concepts to Applications* (Reading, MA: Addison-Wesley)

Carim H M 1988 Bioelectrodes *Encyclopedia of Medical Devices and Instrumentation* ed J G Webster (New York: John Wiley)

Cendes Z J, Shenton D and Shahnasser H 1983 Magnetic field computation using Delaunay triangulation and complementary finite element methods *IEEE Trans. Magnetics* **MAG-19** 2551–4

Cheng K S, Simske S J, Isaacson D, Newell J C and Gisser D G 1989 Errors due to measuring voltage on current-carrying electrodes in electric current computed tomography Personal communication, Dept. of Biomed. Eng., Rensselaer Polytechnic Institute, Troy, NY 12180

Cole K S and Cole R H 1941 Dispersion and absorption in dielectrics *J. Chem. Phys.* **9** 341–51

Condor DC Power Supplies Inc. 1988 *Medical DC Power Supplies* (Oxnard, CA: Condor)

Conte S D and De Boor C 1980 *Elementary Numerical Analysis* (New York: McGraw-Hill)

Conway J 1987 Electrical impedance tomography for thermal monitoring of hyperthermia treatment: an assessment using *in vitro* and *in vivo* measurements *Clin. Phys. Physiol. Meas.* **8 Suppl. A** 141–6

Counts L 1976 Root mean-square *Nonlinear Circuits Handbook* ed D H Sheingold (Norwood, MA: Analog Devices)

Das D P and Webster J G 1980 Defibrillation recovery curves for different electrode materials *IEEE Trans. Biomed. Eng.* **BME-27** 230–3

Dawids S G 1987 Evaluation of applied potential tomography: a clinician's view *Clin. Phys. Physiol. Meas.* **8 Suppl. A** 175–80

Denniston J C and Baker L E 1975 Measurement of urinary bladder emptying using electrical impedance *Med. Biol. Eng.* **13** 305–6

Dines K A and Lytle R J 1981 Analysis of electrical conductivity imaging *Geophysics* **46** 1025–36

Doyle P T and Hill D W 1975 The measurement of residual urine volume by electrical impedance in man *Med. Biol. Eng.* **13** 307–8

Druz W S and Sharp J T 1981 Activity of respiratory muscles in upright and recumbent humans *J. Appl. Physiol.* **51** 1552–61

Duff I S, Erisman A M and Reid J K 1986 *Direct Methods for Sparse Matrices* (New York: Oxford University Press)

Epstein B R and Foster K R 1983 Anisotropy in the dielectric properties of skeletal muscle *Med. Biol. Eng. Comput.* **21** 51–5

Evans W A and Towers M S 1980 Hybrid technique in waveform generation and synthesis *IEE Proc.* G **127** 119–28

EXAR Corporation 1987 *EXAR Databook* (San Jose, CA: EXAR)

Eyuboglu B M, Brown B H and Barber D C 1989 Limitations to SV determination from APT images *Proc. Annu. Int. Conf. IEEE Engineering in Medicine and Biology Society* **11** 442–3

Eyuboglu B M 1989 *Schematics* Personal communication, Duke University, 301 Engineering, Durham, NC 27706

Eyuboglu B M 1988 *Development and application of electrical impedance tomography for thoracic imaging* PhD Thesis, Dept. of Medical Physics and Clinical Engineering, University of Sheffield

Eyuboglu B M, Brown B H, Barber D C and Seagar A D 1987 Localisation of cardiac related impedance changes in the thorax *Clin. Phys. Physiol. Meas.* **8 Suppl. A** 167–73

Fleming D G 1983 Role of home monitoring for infants at risk of SIDS. *Proc. AAMI 18'th Annu. Mtg.* 45

Fricke H and Morse S 1926 The electric capacity of tumors of the breast *J. Cancer. Res.* **10** 340–76

Geddes L A and Baker L E 1989 *Principles of applied biomedical instrumentation* 3rd edn. (New York: John Wiley)

Geddes L and Baker L E 1967 The specific resistance of biological materials—a compendium of data for the biomedical engineer and physiologist *Med. Biol. Eng.* **5** 271–93

George A and Liu J W 1981 *Computer Solution of Large Sparse Positive Definite Systems* (Englewood Cliffs, NJ: Prentice-Hall)

Gibbs N E, Poole W G Jr and Stockmeyer P K 1976 An algorithm for reducing the bandwidth and profile of a sparse matrix *SIAM J. Numer. Anal.* **13** 236–50

Gisser D G, Isaacson D and Newell J C 1987 Current topics in impedance imaging *Clin. Phys. Physiol. Meas.* **8 Suppl. A** 39–46

Gjelsvik A, Aam S and Holten L 1985 Hachtel's augmented matrix method—A rapid method improving numerical stability in power system static state estimation *IEEE Trans. Power Apparatus and Systems* **PAS-104** 2987–92

Goble J and Isaacson D 1989 Optimal current patterns for three-dimensional electric current computed tomography *Proc. Annu. Int. Conf. IEEE Engineering in Medicine and Biology Society* **11** 463–4

Goble J C and Gallagher T D 1988 A distributed architecture for medical instrumentation: an electrical current computed tomograph *Proc. Annu. Int. Conf. IEEE Engineering in Medicine and Biology Society* **10** 285–6

Goldensohn R A and Zablow L 1959 An electrical spirometer *J. Appl. Physiol.* **14** 463–4

Goovaerts H G, de Vries F R, Meijer J H, de Vries P M J M, Donker A J M and Schneider H 1988 Microprocessor-based system for measurement of electrical impedances during haemodialysis and in postoperative care *Med. Biol. Eng. Comput.* **26** 75–80

Gottfried B S and Weisman J 1973 *Introduction to Optimization Theory* (Englewood Cliffs, NJ: Prentice-Hall)

Gould G A, Gugger M, Molloy J and Tsara V 1988 Breathing pattern and eye movement density during REM sleep in humans *Am Rev Respir Dis* **138** 874–7

Griffiths H and Zhang Z 1989 Dual-frequency electrical impedance tomography in vitro and in vivo *Proc. Annu. Int. Conf. IEEE Engineering in Medicine and Biology Society* **11** 476–7

Griffiths H and Ahmed A 1987a A dual-frequency applied potential tomography technique: computer simulations *Clin. Phys. Physiol. Meas.* **8 Suppl. A** 103–7

Griffiths H and Ahmed A 1987b Applied potential tomography for non invasive temperature mapping in hyperthermia *Clin. Phys. Physiol. Meas.* **8 Suppl. A** 147–53

Griffiths H, Antal J and Ahmed A 1985 Non invasive thermometry using applied potential tomography *Strahlentherapie* **161** 534

Hager W W 1988 *Applied Numerical Linear Algebra* (Englewood Cliffs, NJ: Prentice-Hall)

Harris N D, Suggett A J, Barber D C, and Brown B H 1987 Applications of applied potential tomography (APT) in respiratory medicine *Clin. Phys. Physiol. Meas.* **8 Suppl. A** 155–65

Heighway E A and Biddlecombe C S 1982 Two dimensional automatic triangular mesh generation for the finite element electromagnetics package PE2D *IEEE Trans. Magnetics* **MAG-18** 594–8

Henderson R P and Webster J G 1978 An impedance camera for spatially specific measurements of the thorax *IEEE Trans. Biomed. Eng.* **BME-25** 250–4

Henderson R P, Webster J G and Swanson D K 1976 A thoracic electrical impedance camera *Proc. Annu. Conf. Engineering in Medicine and Biology* **18** 322

Hewlett Packard 1988 *Optoelectronics Designer's Catalog, 1988–1989* (Palo Alto, CA: Hewlett Packard)

Hill D W and Thompson F D 1975 The effect of hematocrit on the resistivity of human blood at 37°C and 100 kHz *Med. Biol. Eng.* **13** 182–6

Hu M-Q, Hua P and Webster J G 1987 Measurement error in an electrical impedance tomography system *Proc. Annu. Int. Conf. IEEE Engineering in Medicine and Biology Society* **9** 1425–6

Hua P 1989 *Modeling and reconstruction in electrical impedance tomography* PhD Thesis, Dept. of Electrical and Computer Engineering, Univ. Wisconsin, Madison, WI 53706

Hua P, Webster J G and Tompkins W J 1987 Effect of the measurement method on noise handling and image quality of EIT imaging *Proc. Annu. Int. Conf. IEEE Engineering in Medicine and Biology Society* **9** 1429–30

Hua P, Webster J G and Tompkins W J 1988 A regularised electrical impedance tomography reconstruction algorithm *Clin. Phys. Physiol. Meas.* **9 Suppl. A** 137–41

Hua P, Woo E J, Tompkins W J and Webster J G 1989 An electrical impedance tomograph using compound electrodes *Proc. Annu. Int. Conf. IEEE Engineering in Medicine and Biology Society* **11** 472–3

Hua P 1987 *Electrical impedance tomography in medicine* PhD Preliminary proposal, Dept. of Electrical and Computer Engineering, Univ. Wisconsin, Madison, WI 53706

Huebner K H and Thornton E A 1975 *The Finite Element Method for Engineers* (New York: John Wiley)

Hussain M A, Noble B and Becker B 1989 Computer simulation of an inverse problem for electric current computed tomography using a uniform triangular discretization *Proc. Annu. Int. Conf. IEEE Engineering in Medicine and Biology Society* **11** 448–50

Ider Y Z and Gencer N G 1989 An algorithm for compensating for 3-D effects in electrical impedance tomography *Proc. Annu. Int. Conf. IEEE Engineering in Medicine and Biology Society* **11** 465–6

Ider Y Z, Dorken E, Gencer N G and Koymen H 1988 A dual modality imaging system for impedance tomography with ultrasonically determined boundaries *Proc. Annu. Int. Conf. IEEE Engineering in Medicine and Biology Society* **10** 283–4

Ider Y Z, Altan C, Atalar E and Gencer N G 1987 Electrical impedance imaging system applicable to objects of arbitrary but known boundary *Proc. Annu. Int. Conf. IEEE Engineering in Medicine and Biology Society* **9** 1427–8

Inman Jr. J R, Ryu J and Ward S H 1973 Resistivity inversion *Geophysics* **38** 1088–108

International Electrotechnical Commission 1977 *Safety of Medical Electrical Equipment, Part 1: General Requirements (601-1)* (Geneva: IEC)

Isaacson D 1986 Distinguishability of conductivities by electric current computed tomography *IEEE Trans. Medical Imaging* **MI-5** 91–5

Kanai H, Haeno M and Sakamoto K 1987 Electrical measurement of fluid distribution in legs and arms *Med. Progress through Technol.* **12** 159–70

Kato H, Hiraoka M and Ishida T 1986 An agar phantom for hyperthermia *Med. Phys.* **13** 396–8

Kato H and Ishida T 1987 Development of an agar phantom adaptable for simulation of various tissues in the range 5–40 MHz *Phys. Med. Biol.* **32** 221–6

Kim Y 1982 *A three-dimensional modifiable computer body model and its applications* PhD Thesis, Dept. of Electrical and Computer Engineering, Univ. Wisconsin, Madison, WI 53706

Kim Y, Webster J G and Tompkins W J 1983 Electrical impedance imaging of the thorax *J. Microwave Power* **18** 245–57

Kim Y and Woo H W 1987 A prototype system and reconstruction algorithms for electrical impedance technique in medical body imaging *Clin. Phys. Physiol. Meas.* **8 Suppl. A** 63–70

Kim Y, Woo H W, Brooks T J and Elliott S O 1987 Electrical impedance techniques in imaging: a feasibility study *J. Clin. Eng.* **12** 221–31

King M J 1978 *A four terminal instrumentation system for the measurement of complex bioelectric impedance* MS Thesis, Marquette University, Milwaukee, WI 53233

Kohn R V and Vogelius M 1987 Relaxation of a variational method for impedance computed tomography Dept. of Mathematics, Univ. of Maryland, College Park, MD 20742

Kotre C J 1989 A sensitivity coefficient method for the reconstruction of electrical impedance tomograms *Clin. Phys. Physiol. Meas.* **10** 275–81

Kubicek W G, Kottke F J, Ramos M U, Patterson R P, Witsoe D A, Labree J W, Remole W, Layman T E, Schoening H and Garamela J T 1974 The Minnesota impedance cardiograph—theory and applications *Biomed. Eng.* **9** 410–6

Kubicek W G, Kinnen E and Edin A 1964 Calibration of an impedance pneumograph *J. Appl. Physiol.* **19** 557–60

Kushner R F and Schoeller D A 1986 Estimation of total body water by bioelectric impedance analysis *Am. J. Clin. Nutr.* **44** 417–24

Kulkarni V, Hutchison J M S, Ritchie I K, Chesney R B, Gibson P and Mallard J R 1989 Monitoring fracture healing by impedance imaging *Proc. Annu. Int. Conf. IEEE Engineering in Medicine and Biology Society* **11** 478–9

Liebman F M 1970 Electrical impedance pulse tracings from pulsatile blood flow in rigid tubes and volume restricted vascular beds. *Ann. N.Y. Acad. Sci.* **170** 437–51

Lindholm D A 1983 Automatic triangular mesh generation on surfaces of polyhedra *IEEE Trans. Magnetics* **MAG–19** 2539–42

Lipschultz A 1989 Should U.S. leakage current limits conform to the international standard? *Biomed. Instrum. Technol.* **23** 68–70

Liu W P, Hua P and Webster J G 1988 Three-dimensional reconstruction in electrical impedance tomography *Clin. Phys. Physiol. Meas.* **9 Suppl. A** 131–5

Luedtke A E, Woo H W and Kim Y 1987 Electrical impedance tomography for noninvasive detection of DVT in human calf *Proc. Annu. Int. Conf. IEEE Engineering in Medicine and Biology Society* **9** 1431–2

Lukaski H C, Johnson P E, Bolonchuk W W and Lykken G I 1985 Assessment of fat-free mass using bioelectrical impedance measurements of the body *Am. J. Clin. Nutr.* **41** 810–7

Lytle R J, Bevensee R M and Lager D L 1974 *Three-dimensional subsurface delineation via a novel method for determining the subsurface electrical profile UCRL-51685* Lawrence Livermore Lab., Livermore, CA 94550

Lytle R J and Dines K A 1978 *An impedance camera: A system for determining the spatial variation of electrical conductivity UCRL-52413* Lawrence Livermore Lab., Livermore, CA 94550

Mangnall Y F, Baxter A J, Avill R, Bird N C, Brown B H, Barber D C, Seagar A D, Johnson A G and Read N W 1987 Applied potential tomography: a new non-invasive technique for assessing gastric function *Clin. Phys. Physiol. Meas.* **8 Suppl. A** 119–29

Marquardt D W 1963 An algorithm for least-squares estimation of nonlinear parameters *SIAM J. Appl. Math.* **11** 431–41

McArdle F J, Brown B H and Angel A 1989 Imaging resistivity changes of the adult brain during the cardiac cycle *Proc. Annu. Int. Conf. IEEE Engineering in Medicine and Biology Society* **11** 480–1

McClelland G R and Sutton J A 1985 Epigastric impedance: a non invasive method for the assessment of gastric emptying and motility *Gut* **26** 607–14

McDougall D and Shizgal H M 1986 Body composition measurements from whole body resistance and reactance *Surgical Forum* **37** 42–4

Mineo B A 1986 A portable non invasive ultrasonic bladder sensor for incontinence *Proc. Annu. Int. Conf. IEEE Engineering in Medicine and Biology Society* **8** 1864–7

Murai T and Kagawa Y 1985 Electrical impedance computed tomography based on a finite element model *IEEE Trans. Biomed. Eng.* **BME-32** 177–84

Murphy D, Burton P, Coombs R, Tarassenko L and Rolfe P 1987 Impedance imaging in the newborn *Clin. Phys. Physiol. Meas.* **8 Suppl. A** 131–40

Murphy D and Rolfe P 1988 Aspects of instrumentation design for impedance imaging *Clin. Phys. Physiol. Meas.* **9 Suppl. A** 5–14

Nakayama K, Yagi W and Yagi S 1981 Fundamental study on electrical impedance CT algorithm utilizing sensitivity theorem on impedance plethsmography *Proc. 5th Int. Conf. on Electrical Bio-impedance (ICEBI)* 99–102

National Fire Protection Association 1987 *Health Care Facilities (ANSI/NFPA 99-1987)* (Quincy, MA: NFPA)

Newell J C, Gisser D G and Isaacson D 1988 An electric current tomograph *IEEE Trans. Biomed. Eng.* **35** 828–33

Newman M R 1978 Biopotential amplifiers *Medical Instrumentation: Application and Design* ed J G Webster (Boston, MA: Houghton Mifflin)

Nowicki D J and Webster J G 1989 A one op-amp current source for electrical impedance tomography *Proc. Annu. Int. Conf. IEEE Engineering in Medicine and Biology Society* **11** 457–8

Nyboer J, Bagno S, Barnett A and Halsey R H 1950 Radiocardiograms: Electrical impedance changes of the heart in relation to electrocardiograms and heart sounds *J. Clin. Invest.* **19** 963

Pallas-Areny R 1989 *Schematics* Personal communication, Departamento de Ingenieria Electronica, Division de Instrumentacion y Bioingenieria, U.P.C., 08080 Barcelona, Spain

Patterson R, Ranganathan C, Engel R and Berkseth R 1988 Measurement of body fluid volume change using multisite impedance measurements *Med. Biol. Eng. Comp.* **26** 33–7

Pethig R 1979 *Dielectric and Electric Properties of Biological Materials* (Chichester: John Wiley)

Pethig R 1984 Dielectric properties of biological materials: biophysical and medical applications *IEEE Trans. Elec. Insulation* **EI-19** 453–74

Pico Electronics Inc. 1988 *Pico Catalog 2014A* (Mt. Vernon, NY: Pico Electronics Inc.)

Pilkington T, Eyuboglu M and Wolf P 1989 Utilization of esophageal reference electrode to enhance impedance imaging *Proc. Annu. Int. Conf. IEEE Engineering in Medicine and Biology Society* **11** 482

Plonsey R and Collin R 1977 Electrode guarding in electrical impedance measurements of physiological systems—a critique *Med. Biol. Eng. Comp.* **15** 519–27

Pomerantz M, Baumgartner R, Lauridson J and Eiseman B 1969 Transthoracic electrical impedance for the early detection of pulmonary edema *Surgery* **66** 260–8

Porter J M and Swain I D 1987 Measurement of cardiac output by electrical impedance plethysmography *J. Biomed. Eng.* **9** 222–31

Powell H M, Barber D C and Freeston I L 1987 Impedance imaging using linear electrode arrays *Clin. Phys. Physiol. Meas.* **8 Suppl. A** 109–18

Powell H M, Barber D C and Freeston I L 1985 Impedance imaging using a linear electrode array *Proc. IEE Int. Conf. on Electric and Magnetic Fields in Medicine and Biology* 88–92

Railton R, Fischer J, Mitchell I and Barclay R P C 1983 Long-term respiration monitoring in infants—a comparison of impedance and pressure capsule monitors *Clin. Phys. Physiol. Meas.* **4** 91–4

Reddy G N and Saha S 1984 Electrical and dielectric properties of wet bone as a function of frequency *IEEE Trans. Biomed. Eng.* **BME-31** 296–302

Rosell J, Riu P and Pallas-Areny R 1989 A parallel data acquisition system for electrical impedance tomography *Proc. Annu. Int. Conf. IEEE Engineering in Medicine and Biology Society* **11** 459–60

Rosell J, Colominas J, Riu P, Pallas R and Webster J G 1988a Skin impedance from 1 Hz to 1 MHz *IEEE Trans. Biomed. Eng.* **35** 649–651

Rosell J, Murphy P, Pallas R and Rolfe P 1988b Analysis and assessment of errors in a parallel data acquisition system for electrical impedance tomography *Clin. Phys. Physiol. Meas.* **9 Suppl. A** 93–99

Rosenfeld A and Kak A C 1982 *Digital Picture Processing* (New York: Academic Press)

Roy K K and Rao K P 1977 Limiting depth of detection in line electrode systems *Geophys. Pros.* **25** 758–67

Rush S, Abildskov J A and McFee R 1963 Resistivity of body tissues at low frequencies *Circ. Res.* **12** 40–50

Sabonnadiere J C and Coulomb J L 1987 *Finite Element Methods in CAD* (New York: Springer-Verlag)

Sahakian A V, Tompkins W J and Webster J G 1985 Electrode motion artifacts in electrical impedance pneumography *IEEE Trans. Biomed. Eng.* **BME-32** 449–51

Sakamoto K, Yorkey T J and Webster J G 1987 Some physical results from an impedance camera *Clin. Phys. Physiol. Meas.* **8 Suppl. A** 71–6

Sato N and Tinney W F 1963 Techniques for exploiting the sparsity of the network admittance matrix *IEEE Trans. Power Apparatus and Systems* **PAS-82** 944–9

Schwan H P 1957 Electrical properties of tissue and cell suspensions *Adv. Biol. Med. Phys.* **5** 147–209

Schwan H P and Kay C F 1956 Specific resistance of body tissues *Circ. Res.* **4** 644–70

Seagar A D, Barber D C and Brown B H 1987 Theoretical limits to sensitivity and resolution in impedance imaging *Clin. Phys. Physiol. Meas.* **8 Suppl. A** 13–31

Seagar A and Bates R 1985 Full-wave computed tomography. Part 4: Low-frequency electric current CT *IEE Proc.* A **132** 455–66

Seagar A, Yeo M and Bates R 1984 Full-wave computed tomography. Part 2: Resolution limits *IEE Proc.* A **131** 612–22

Sequent Computer Systems Inc. 1987 *Sequent Guide to Parallel Programming* (San Jose, CA: Sequent Computer Systems Inc.)

Skidmore R, Evans J M, Jenkins D and Wells P N T 1987 A data collection system for gathering electrical impedance measurements from the human breast *Clin. Phys. Physiol. Meas.* **8 Suppl. A** 99–102

Smith R W M, Freeston I L and Brown B H 1989 Digital demodulation for electrical impedance imaging *Proc. Annu. Int. Conf. IEEE Engineering in Medicine and Biology Society* **11** 1744–5

Stein I M 1979 Patterns of pediatric pneumogram *Med. Instrum.* **13** 177–80

Stuchly M A and Stuchly S S 1984 Electrical properties of biological substance *Biological Effects and Medical Applications of Electromagnetic Fields* ed O P Ghandi (New York: Academic Press)

Swanson D K 1976 *Measurement errors and the origin of electrical impedance changes in the limb* PhD Thesis, Dept. Electrical and Computer Eng., Univ. Wisconsin, Madison, WI 53706

Tarassenko L, Pidcock M K, Murphy D F and Rolfe P 1985 The development of impedance imaging techniques for use in the newborn at risk of intra-ventricular hemorrhage *Proc. IEE Int. Conf. on Electric and Magnetic Fields in Medicine and Biology* 83–7

Tasto M and Schomberg H 1978 Object reconstruction from projections and some non-linear extensions *Pattern Recognition and Signal Processing* ed C H Chen (Alphen aan den Rijn: Sijthoff & Noordhoff)

Telford W M, Geldart L P, Sheriff R E and Key D A 1976 *Applied Geophysics—Resistivity Methods* (Cambridge: Cambridge University Press)

Tinney W F, Brandwajin V and Chan S M 1985 Sparse vector methods *IEEE Trans. Power Apparatus and Systems* **PAS-104** 295–301

Tinney W F and Walker J W 1967 Direct solutions of sparse network equations by optimally ordered triangular factorization *Proc. IEEE* **55** 1801–9

Tobey G E, Graeme J G and Huelsman L P 1971 *Operational Amplifiers: Design and Applications* (New York: McGraw-Hill)

Tong P and Rossettos J N 1977 *Finite Element Method: Basic Technique and Implementation* (Cambridge, MA: MIT Press)

Towers M S 1982 Programmable waveform generator using linear interpolation with multiplying D/A convertors *IEE Proc.* G **129** 18–25

Underwriters Laboratories 1976 *Medical and Dental Equipment (UL544)* (Melville, NY: Underwriters Laboratories)

Van der Walt P W 1981 A Wien-bridge oscillator with high-amplitude stability *IEEE Trans. Instr. Meas.* **IM-30** 292–4

Volpe J J 1981 Current methods in neonatal medicine *N. Eng. J. Med.* **304** 886–91

Warburton D, Stark A R and Taeusch H W 1977 Apnea monitor failure in infants with upper airway obstruction *Pediatrics* **60** 742–4

Webster J G 1978a Amplifiers and signal processing *Medical Instrumentation: Application and Design* ed J G Webster (Boston: Houghton Mifflin)

Webster J G 1978b Measurement of flow and volume of blood *Medical Instrumentation: Application and Design* ed J G Webster (Boston: Houghton Mifflin)

Wexler A 1988 Electrical impedance imaging in two and three dimensions *Clin. Phys. Physiol. Meas.* **9 Suppl. A** 29–33

Wexler A, Fry B and Neuman M R 1985 Impedance-computed tomography algorithm and system *Appl. Optics* **24** 3985–92

Wiley J D and Webster J G 1982 Distributed equivalent circuit models for circular dispersive electrodes *IEEE Trans. Biomed. Eng.* **BME-29** 385–9

Winfield D L, Trachtman L H and Rouse D J 1988 Space solutions for the earthbound medical problems *SOMA* **2** 42–8

Wojslaw C F and Moustakas E A 1986 *Operational Amplifiers* (New York: John Wiley)

Woo E J, Hua P, Tompkins W J and Webster J G 1989 32-electrode electrical impedance tomograph—software design and static images *Proc. Annu. Int. Conf. IEEE Engineering in Medicine and Biology Society* **11** 455–6

Woo E J, Hua P, Tompkins W J and Webster J G 1988 A finite element model with node renumbering for adaptive impedance imaging *Proc. Annu. Int. Conf. IEEE Engineering in Medicine and Biology Society* **10** 277–8

Yamamoto T and Yamamoto Y 1976a Electrical properties of the epidermal stratum corneum *Med. Biol. Eng.* **14** 151–8

Yamamoto T and Yamamoto Y 1976b Dielectric constant and resistivity of epidermal stratum corneum *Med. Biol. Eng.* **14** 494–9

Yorkey T 1986 *Comparing reconstruction methods for electrical impedance tomography* PhD Thesis, Dept. of Electrical and Computer Eng., Univ. Wisconsin, Madison, WI 53706

Yorkey T J, Webster J G and Tompkins W J 1985 Errors caused by contact impedance in impedance imaging *Proc. Annu. Int. Conf. IEEE Engineering in Medicine and Biology Society* **7** 632–7

Yorkey T J, Webster J G and Tompkins W J 1986 An optimal impedance tomographic reconstruction algorithm *Proc. Annu. Int. Conf. IEEE Engineering in Medicine and Biology Society* **8** 339–42

Yorkey T J, Webster J G and Tompkins W J 1987a Comparing reconstruction algorithms for electrical impedance tomography *IEEE Trans. Biomed. Eng.* **BME-34** 843–52

Yorkey T J, Webster J G and Tompkins W J 1987b An improved perturbation technique for electrical impedance imaging with some criticisms *IEEE Trans. Biomed. Eng.* **BME-34** 898–901

Zheng E, Shao S and Webster J G 1984 Impedance of skeletal muscle from 1 Hz to 1 MHz *IEEE Trans. Biomed. Eng.* **BME-31** 477–81

Index